SalonOvations'
Advanced Skin Care
Handbook

SalonOvations'
Advanced Skin Care
Handbook

Lia Schorr
with Shari Sims

SalonOvations
(A Division of Milady Publishing Company)

Delmar Publishers' Online Services

To access Delmar on the World Wide Web, point your browser to:

http://www.delmar.com/delmar.html

To access through Gopher: gopher://gopher.delmar.com

(Delmar Online is part of "thomson.com", an Internet site with information on
more than 30 publishers of the International Thomson Publishing organization.)

For information on our products and services:

email: info@delmar.com

or call 800-347-7707

Credits

Publisher: Catherine Frangie
Senior Developmental Editor: Laura V. Miller
Developmental Editor: Annette L. Danaher
Senior Art/Design Supervisor: Susan C. Mathews
Production Manager: John Mickelbank
Project Editor: Annette L. Danaher

Cover Design by: design M design W
Cover Photo by: Mariko Abe/Photonica

© 1994 SalonOvations
(A Division of Milady Publishing Company)

For information address:
SalonOvations
(A Division of Milady Publishing Company)
3 Columbia Circle, Box 12519
Albany, NY 12212-2519

Printed in the United States of America
Printed and Distributed simultaneously in Canada

2 3 4 5 6 7 8 9 10 XXX 00 99 98 97 96

Library of Congress Cataloging-in-Publication Data

Schorr, Lia.
  SalonOvations' advanced skin care handbook / Lia Schorr with Shari Sims.
    p.   cm.   Includes glossary/index.
  ISBN 1-56253-045-3
  1. Beauty culture. 2. Skin—Care and hygiene. I. Sims, Shari
Miller. II. Title.
TT958.S36   1994
646.7'26—dc20   93-44635
                                                          CIP

DEDICATION

To my daughter Segaal, who continues to bring pleasure and magic into my life and allows me the time and space to complete my work

and

To any person who chooses to be a part of the exciting industry of beauty—to a student, business owner, salon employee, or anyone interested in the art and science of this industry

Contents

Preface

Skin care (also known as esthetics or cosmetology) has been a basic for European women for hundreds of years, both at home and as done by professionals in spas and salons. Yet in America it has only recently, within the past decade or so, become a subject of interest to the masses. Forty years ago, when the first American salon opened for business, only the wealthy thought they could afford this type of service. That is no longer the case. Today, women and men alike are spending tremendous sums on the care and preservation of their skin— a total of *$6 billion* in 1992 alone, according to market researchers at Kline & Co. The numbers of salons catering to skin care clients has also grown, to roughly 8,000 across the United States at this time.

Of course, specialized salons aren't the only place to find skin care professionals at work. You'll find them in the growing numbers of spas across the country, behind department-store counters, and in the executive suites of cosmetic companies. According to *Modern Salon* magazine's 1992 Salon Owner Survey Report, 40 percent of hair salons now also offer skin care services, with 44 percent of those salons having a trained skin care specialist on staff. In fact, the 1992 survey showed that "skin care is the fastest growing area of the professional beauty industry," according to an article in the December 1992 issue of the magazine.

The opportunities to learn, grow, and prosper within this field are constantly expanding. Consider these statements from a July 12, 1993, article in the *New York Times*:

> Indeed, at a time when employment in many blue- and white-collar fields continues to sputter, there is strong demand for cosmetologists. Currently, some 40,000 jobs are estimated to be unfilled, and (a) survey... indicated that half of the nation's salons had a hard time finding new employees.

Few other professions are as wide open as this one, or as accepting of new ideas and enthusiasm.

But as with any profession, new ideas aren't the only ingredients needed for success. You need a grounding in the facts—the science and the practice of skin care that allows you to experiment and improve upon your experience. That's where this book comes in. It is intended to guide you from the beginning stages of esthetics to more specialized positions on up through salon manager to salon owner, and it is written by someone who herself worked her way up through those very stages. This book was written, in part, for a very practical reason: When I decided to open a school of esthetics to share my knowledge with others, I was surprised to find, in a visit to the library, how little written material there was specifically on the subject of professional skin care. There are lots of books for the public, so-called beauty books and health and fitness books, but very few that are targeted specifically to the skin care profession. And the best of these books was written fifteen years ago, since which time many changes have occurred.

Another prime reason for writing this book is to share the specialness of the role of an esthetician. Few other careers give one the chance to represent beauty and esthetics within the world, to act as a role model, to nurture clients' meditative sides, to broaden their philosophies, to teach the how-tos of makeup and skin care, to provide information that is personally helpful, and to help others literally feel better about themselves. Despite the hype that is all around us, you won't find many gimmicks or tricks in these pages; what you will find is an honest, common-sense approach based on caring for each individual client. After twenty-six years in the business, sixteen of them in running my own shop, that's what I have found is most crucial to success: honesty, human relations, and caring—not puffery or falsely inflated promises. Some information may seem very basic; however, the most basic is often the most overlooked. I mention these topics as *tips* for running a successful business—they have been essential in my personal experiences.

In fact, this book is intended to help those who, whether just starting out in the field or hoping to advance themselves, want to offer the most innovative approaches to solving skin care problems. This book is for you if you are interested in what is newest and most valuable, most scientific, most realistic, and most beneficial, for your clients and yourself. Too often, consumers and cosmetologists alike are taken in by hyped-up sales pitches for treatments or products that are ineffective at best, or sometimes even dangerous. One goal of this book is to help you arm yourself with the type of solid information that will help you resist such false expectations.

Many subjects are covered in this book—too many, in fact, for you to absorb all at once. Consider this a handbook of skin care information to dip into when you are in need of specific answers, whether on purchasing salon equipment, treating acne-prone teenage skin, advising a client how to take care of her complexion at home, or offering "special" facials for sensitive, aging, or dry skin. This is a textbook for skin care advancement, a wonderful gift to give someone in the industry, a student, a professional in the self-image or fashion business, or someone who is thinking of opening or has opened her/his own salon. It is based on the beliefs that the best way to enhance the skin care profession is to become as educated as possible, and that the goal of any professional should be to keep learning throughout one's career.

A WORD ABOUT TRAINING

In any field, you are only as good as what you know, and the way to be sure that your knowledge base is strong is to study on your own and attend a respected school. Beware of any institution that does not have experienced skin care professionals on the staff. In some states, hairdressing and skin care licensing overlap, but you want to be sure that the skin-oriented portion of your education is directed by those who have hands-on experience in the skin care field. Don't overlook the importance of continuing education. Take advantage of seminars, meetings, and conferences in your area.

USING THIS BOOK TO YOUR ADVANTAGE

Too often, we read something once and then put it away. But this book is meant to help you now, with gaining immediate knowledge, and in the future, when specific needs arise within your professional life. It is organized in a way that will carry you through the various steps of your career, from beginning as an esthetician, to interviewing new clients and offering them basic facials, to giving more advanced facial and body treatments and specialized procedures (such as ionic facials, body rubs, or aromatherapy), and finishing with the kinds of challenges that confront a salon manager and owner, from advertising and public relations to selecting a site for and designing one's own salon.

Obviously, you may not need all this information right now, this very day. But you will want to have it handy as soon as it's required, and this book is set up to make it as easy as possible to get the information you need. Many people shared their knowledge with me through the years to help me get to where I am today; it is my hope that by organizing this book in as straightforward a manner as possible, I will make it possible for my colleagues and peers to benefit from my experience, learn from my mistakes, and help the skin care field grow to an ever more respected and valuable profession.

Acknowledgments

I would like to thank the skin care industry for making me feel alive and challenged. Being a part of such an exciting industry helped me grow, share, work, and go farther than I ever expected.

I would also like to thank Shari Miller Sims for saying yes, after two years of my effort, and writing this book with me. It was worth it taking the time to persuade you. I couldn't have done it without you. Your talent at writing, knowledge, and intelligence are behind every word in this book. You are my perfect match. Thank you for your friendship and for choosing me as a coauthor for a third time.

To Cathy Frangie, who accepted this proposal, I would also like to extend my appreciation. Without her, the dream of this book would not have come true. The taste, trust, and respect she provided to Shari and me made it special to work on this book.

In closing, I would like to express my appreciation to everyone who stood behind me during all the years since I started my business—friends, clients, employees, and especially members of the press, who believe in my knowledge and let me bring needed information on skin care to their audiences.

Thank you to the following professionals for their expertise and very helpful input while reviewing this manuscript:

Anna Caldarelli
Renee Poignard
Joseph Anthony
Mark Lees
Sabra Haywood
Carol Phillips

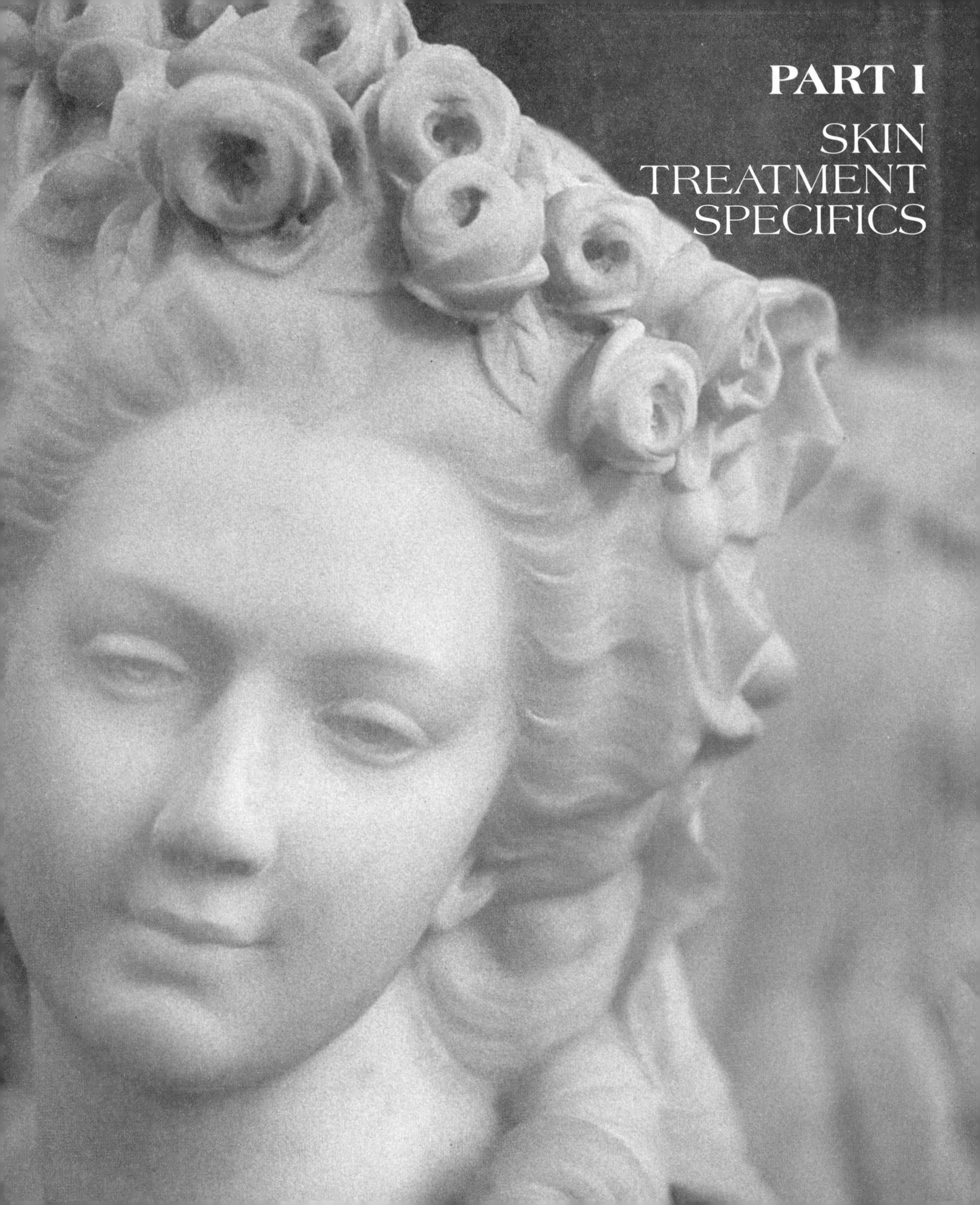

CHAPTER 1

Skin Basics:
Understanding How the Skin Works

The skin is the body's largest and most complex organ, but it is also the one people take most for granted. Caring for the skin is a pleasure and a responsibility. You can give your clients the best possible care by understanding how the skin works from the inside out. In this chapter, you will find out about:

- skin physiology and metabolism: the basic building blocks of young, healthy skin
- why skin needs to be cared for and nurtured
- women versus men: skin similarities and differences
- the influence of genetics and ethnic background
- the effects of stress and aging.

THE SKIN'S INNER STRUCTURE

It is important for every esthetician to know about the structure of the skin, because the greater your understanding, the greater the knowledge you can share with and use for your clients. All body tissues are made up of individual cells filled with proto-plasm, a colorless, jelly-like substance in which complex molecules, among other things, are present. Although cells can be seen only under high-powered microscopes, the skin care products of the modern age do their jobs by penetrating into these microscopic structures.

Cells within the body are found in groups called **tissue**, with each kind of tissue carrying out a specific function. The five key types of tissue found in the human body are:

1. **Connective Tissue** This type of tissue serves to support, protect, and bind together other tissues of the body. Bone, cartilage, ligaments, tendons, and fat are examples of connective tissue.

2. **Muscle Tissue** These strong groups of cells contract and move various parts of the body. Muscles help form facial

expressions, help a Rockette kick up her legs, and help an artist draw the finest of lines within a painting.

3. **Nerve Tissue** These cell groups are the body's communication system, carrying messages to and from the brain and controlling and coordinating all body functions.

4. **Epithelial Tissue** This specialized kind of tissue acts as a protective covering on body surfaces, such as the skin, mucous membranes, glands, and linings of the heart, digestive, and respiratory organs.

5. **Liquid Tissue** This tissue carries food, waste products, and hormones by means of the blood and lymph supply.

No matter what the type of body tissue, moisture is essential to its health—moisture absorbed from the air and taken in through foods and liquids. Without the proper moisture balance, the body cannot carry out its daily functions.

The skin itself has several important functions that it must perform every day. These include:

- acting as a shield to protect internal organs against invasion by foreign substances or damage from the radiation of the sun

- housing the sense organs that allow us to react to pleasure and danger

- regulating internal body temperature

- storehousing needed nutrients

- helping to eliminate waste products.

If you have any doubt that the skin is called upon to perform many functions, consider this: In an average square inch of skin, there are approximately 20 blood vessels, 65 hairs, 100 or more oil glands, 650 or more sweat glands (to act as both thermostats and waste removers), 28 nerves, 13 sense receptors for cold, 78 heat sensors, and 1,300 sensors to respond to touch, whether pleasurable or painful. Viewed in this way, it's easy to see why the skin is such a marvel.

SKIN LAYERS

The skin is made up of three main layers. The outermost, which is the only one we can see, is the **epidermis**; next comes the inner, thicker layer, called the **dermis**; and under that is the **subcutaneous** layer, made up primarily of cushiony fat. Each layer varies in thickness depending on which part of the body it covers—and each has a very distinct function. (**Fig. 1.1**)

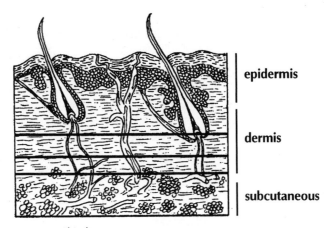

Fig. 1.1. Skin layers.

The Epidermis

The part of the skin that can be seen is the epidermis—or, to be more precise, its outermost layer of dead skin cells or keratin. These flat, "horny" cells are made up of about 80 percent protein (or keratin) and barely 20 percent water, as opposed to the 70 percent water that makes up internal living cells. The thickness of the keratin varies; for example, it is thicker in men than women and in certain areas (such as the knees) than others (e.g., the paper-thin eyelids). One thing is certain, though: a healthy epidermis waterproofs the body and helps to destroy certain microorganisms through its naturally acidic pH.

The outermost layer of the epidermis can be smooth and soft or rough and dry. What determines the difference is climate (how much moisture the air robs from the skin), overall health, and the care that is taken of the skin. Skin cells live an average of twenty-four to thirty days, so once a month, on average, this outermost layer is shed in favor of new cells. In young, smooth, well-cared-for skin, this shedding is virtually invisible, although that can change with sun damage, dryness, and aging.

The deepest layer of the epidermis, called the **basal layer**, is made up of cells that are constantly dividing and pushing their way upward. The cells of this layer are also called into play when the skin is injured, such as by a scrape. The basal layer responds by speeding up the cell reproduction process to replace damaged cells with healthy new ones.

Some of the cells in this layer are also specialized **melanocytes**, which produce the pigment (or **melanin**) that gives skin its natural coloration. Everyone, regardless of skin color or sex, has the same number of melanocytes, but the size of the granules and the amount of pigment they produce are genetically determined. Melanocytes are derived from nerve tissue and are the producers of the skin's own natural sunscreen.

The Dermis

Dermatologists call this layer the "true skin" because it contains the collagen fibers that give the skin its structure and shape, along with the blood vessels, lymph vessels, nerves, hair follicle "roots," and sweat and sebaceous glands. The dermis nourishes the basal layer of the epidermis.

To keep skin in tiptop shape, the dermis must be full, soft, and elastic. Most movements of the body, even just forming a smile, require some stretching or wrinkling of the skin. A healthy dermis enables the body to do this and return to its natural shape.

The networks of blood vessels within the dermis give the skin its warmth and tone. Constriction of these blood vessels, whether due to illness, smoking, or stress, can sap the skin of its healthy-looking color.

Subcutaneous Tissue

The dermis is attached to fatty tissue with strong collagen fibers. This fatty tissue varies in thickness according to certain body areas as well as the sex, age, and weight of the individual. It is a direct lesson that not all fat is bad; without any fat the skin could not have contour and shape, and the body could not possibly retain its steady internal temperature.

MAINTAINING SKIN HEALTH

Fresh air, exercise, adequate vitamin intake, and a balanced diet are still the best possible treatments for the skin. But the fact is that many habits of modern life counteract these needs. People spend days on end cooped up indoors in offices with stale, recirculated air; they rarely get enough physical activity; they eat on the run—and eat too much as often as too little. When Americans do get outdoors, they tend to overdo it, exposing their skin to the most damaging rays of the sun.

That's why professional skin care consultations can be so valuable. They give our clients the opportunity to learn about the steps they can take to make the most of their skin's health. It's a time to focus on oneself for a busy person and to focus on the changes that can provide lasting benefits, such as using sunscreens, thoroughly cleansing the skin before bedtime, and having regular skin cleanings to prevent clogged pores.

One of the most common questions clients ask about the physiology of the skin is whether the pores can be "closed" after they have enlarged. Pores are not like doors that can be opened and closed at will. Dead skin cells, makeup, and pollution all collect within the pores, stretching the openings. When this cellular debris is properly removed—and this means by the gentle professional extraction method, not at-home picking and squeezing—the pore walls do usually come back together a bit. Although the pores can't literally be shrunk, cleansing them makes them much less obvious. Ironically, many clients ask these questions after they have attempted at-home cleaning that has made their pores more, rather than less, obvious by producing microscopic bruising in the sensitive skin cells around and within the pore openings.

Another common question is whether the skin "breathes." Though it does not do so in the same way that the lungs do, it is true that the skin takes in oxygen and releases carbon dioxide. According to one estimate, roughly 1 percent of the carbon dioxide released by the body is given off through the skin. Increasing the skin's oxygen level is a goal of many skin treatments. There is an important lesson in the unfortunate case in which the use of gold paint to completely coat the body resulted in death by asphyxiation, because the body could not get enough oxygen in through the skin.

GENDER AND THE SKIN: MORE THE SAME THAN DIFFERENT

Many people naturally assume that women's skin is totally different from men's skin, but in fact they are more alike than not. The biggest influences on skin's condition are still its degree of oiliness or dryness and how much or how little sun damage one gets.

That said, it is true that men's skin is naturally a bit thicker than women's. Also, the fact that men shave packs a double effect. One good side effect is that shaving naturally sloughs off dead surface cells. At the other extreme, though, shaving can be hard on sensitive skin—and many men don't do much to help their complexions deal with the daily or every-other-day assault that shaving can be. Men's skin also doesn't vary quite as much as women's, because they don't undergo the monthly hormonal swings involved in menstruation or the hormonal upheavals of pregnancy and menopause.

Where men and women often differ is in what could be called their knowledge gaps about their skin. The biggest danger to many a man's skin in America is a lack of awareness about taking care of his complexion. The biggest danger to women's skin in this country, however, is often overtreating, overdoing, and overwhelming the skin with too many products, too much makeup, and too much manipulation.

THE POWER OF OUR GENES: HEREDITY AND THE SKIN

Although climate, environment, and how each person cares for the skin make a big difference in skin health and appearance, the starting point is, quite literally, the skin one is born with. One's skin, in many ways, reflects one's heritage. As skin care professionals, we need to be sensitive to ethnic differences in skin types while being aware that stereotyping, in any field, can be seen as demeaning. It's not uncommon, after all, for clients today to be of mixed heritage and for a skin type to reflect a melting-pot genetic heritage. That doesn't preclude the fact, however, that certain skin characteristics usually go along with the four major groups in America: Caucasian, Black, Hispanic, and Asian. Following are some general observations based on contact with hundreds of clients over the years. As with all generalizations, they are meant only as overall guidelines; not all of the factors will apply to everyone. A firsthand view of a client's skin through the magnifying lens is still the best guide to what that individual's skin requires.

Caucasian Skin

Caucasian skin can be subdivided into two basic groups: fair (Nordic/British) and olive (or Mediterranean). Fair skin is light-colored, thin-textured, and highly vulnerable to dryness, broken capillaries, and environmental damage from wind and sun. It often reddens immediately upon contact with an irritant.

Olive Skin

Olive skin tends to be oilier and more prone to blackheads, but it has slightly more natural protection against sunburn and windburn as a result of its darker pigment. Darker toned complexions can scar more easily from acne or injury.

Black Skin

Black skin contains a higher concentration of melanin in its cells than Caucasian skin but, contrary to popular belief, is not at all immune to the hazards of sun-induced aging and skin cancer. Roughly 7 percent of the clientele in a typical salon is Black. "Black" skin ranges in coloration from pale brown to dark ebony, and the varieties of skin tendencies match this range. One common misconception is that Black skin is oily. The fact is that 5 percent of Black clients have extremely dry complexions, which often appear as ashy or gray-looking patches. Persons of mixed racial backgrounds can have skin ranging from the reddish undertones of Native Americans to the brown/gray pigmentation of Oriental Indians. Because pigment can sometimes mask surface problems, it's crucial to pay attention to what you see when you look at the skin under the magnifying light, not to make preconceptions your guide.

Hispanic Skin

Hispanic skin is rarely dry, but it also isn't always oily. Very often, it's a combination of dry-to-normal areas with oily patches. Although we tend to think of Hispanic skin as olive skin, it can range in coloration from olive to brown, and it too needs to be protected from the sun's damaging rays. The common fashion among many women of Hispanic heritage of using a greater-than-average amount of makeup can sometimes aggravate breakouts of blackheads or acne-type lesions.

Asian Skin

Asian skin can range from pale yellow to deeper brown. In general, this skin type is highly sensitive; although acne is not overly common, once the skin becomes acne- or blemish-prone, it tends to heal very slowly over periods of weeks rather than days. You may find that Asian men who suffer nicks and cuts during shaving heal more slowly than Caucasian men.

GROWING UP WITH OUR SKINS: CHANGES THROUGH THE YEARS

It's not uncommon for a skin care salon to have clients of a wide range of ethnic backgrounds and ages, because attention to appearance starts young today—and, let's face it, skin problems often first develop in the teens. The key reason is the effect of so-called raging hormones. The reality is that, whether or not they rage, **hormones** have an effect on the skin. They can upset or balance the skin's condition, producing the overactive sweat glands of nervousness or the allergy-like rashes of stress. Acne is acknowledged by almost all medical authorities to have a hormonal component; although no one can quite agree on the exact mechanism, there's no question that the skin is influenced by hormones.

The most extreme problems (namely **cystic acne**, **psoriasis**, **eczema**, and **rashes**) are probably best dealt with by medical professionals. The one area a skin care specialist can influence is the effect of stress, which tends to exacerbate the skin's tendencies, causing increased dryness for someone with a dry complexion and more breakouts for someone with minor blackheads or blemishes. In creating a calming atmosphere and attitude, a salon facial can do a lot to defuse tension, helping a client's attitude and complexion. That oasis of calm applies at any age.

The Teen Years

Aside from the emotional upheaval the teen years often produce, it's the prime age for hormonally aggravated acne. Poor eating habits, too much sun, and picking at the skin often irritate an already overactive complexion. Yet this is also the age when an esthetician can teach young clients their most important skin care lessons for life—if you can just get them into the salon for that education!

Many teenagers don't understand that cleansing the skin also means keeping their hair clean, their fingers clean, and their clothes clean, because dirt and bacteria on all of these can be transferred to the skin. Blackheads and whiteheads shouldn't be self-cleaned, and some severe blemishes really require a dermatologist's care to avoid later scarring.

Many teens are brought to a skin care salon by their parents, but that doesn't mean that regular visits are necessary. Once a week may be needed at first to establish a good skin care regimen, but once a month or every few months might be more appropriate later on. At many salons, a special discount is given to teenagers to acknowledge the reality of the high cost of this kind of professional care (and some salons even continue this type of discount plan for college students and/or their twenty-something clients).

The Twenties

The twenties are usually a great time for the skin. Teen break-outs are often subsiding (if they've been taken care of properly) and the buoyant spirits of young persons striking out on their own in the work world are reflected in the natural glow of their complexions. It's the age when many people first become aware of taking care of their complexions. Young men going to an office may be shaving daily for the first time in their lives, while young women are more likely to begin wearing makeup on an everyday basis even if they didn't during their student years.

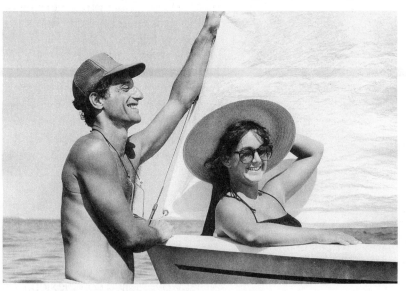

Fig. 1.2. Take precautions when in the sun.

There are important lessons to be learned at this stage. First and foremost is the importance of taking precautions when out in the sun—always wearing sunscreen and never baking to a deep, dark tan. Sun damage may be invisible at this age, but the cumulative toll is starting to make its mark by the late twenties, often when the very first tiny lines begin to appear. (**Fig. 1.2**) Women need to remember not to wear makeup when

SPOTLIGHT
....

The fifteen-year-old girl who walked into my salon with her mother looked older than her age at first glance (too much makeup, it turned out) but was terribly insecure once we sat down to talk. Her mother proceeded to tell me, "Money is no object; just clear up my daughter's skin, please." I assured the woman that I would do whatever I could and then examined her daughter's skin under the magnifying light, where I saw the telltale signs of a teenager picking at and "popping" her own pimples in a misguided effort to clear up her skin.

At this point, I asked the mother if she could please take a seat in the waiting room so that I could give her daughter a facial geared to her skin type. Comfortably settled with a cup of coffee and a magazine, the woman entrusted her daughter to my care. Freed of her mother's presence, the teenager then told me that sometimes her mother actually helped her clean her skin, "getting at" the pimples she herself left behind. They once went to a dermatologist who prescribed an antibiotic, but the girl had a bad reaction to it (she didn't tell me what) and they never went back.

I gave her a gentle but thorough skin cleansing, followed by an antibacterial aloe/calamine mask. I then advised her that if she would come back twice a week for facials for a while, and agree not to wear any makeup until her skin had cleared, I thought we could make a big difference in two months or so.

The daughter and her mother agreed. And the results, just six weeks later, were surprising even to me. Her skin looked fresher and healthier, and the marks left by too much at-home "surgery" were lighter and much less noticeable. At the six-week mark, after so much progress had been made, we picked out some new makeup colors for her to use and went over their application together. The girl told me she'd be "in debt to [me] for life."

In fact, that once-scared teenager is still my client thirteen years later. She no longer needs to come so often, of course, but has yet to skip an appointment except when business travel or vacations interrupt. She is equally special to me as someone whom I have watched grow and mature into a lovely person who now takes pride in herself and her own appearance and has a sense of self-image that goes much deeper than what she looks like. These are the kinds of rewards that taking the time to educate your clients can create.

exercising, because it can clog the pores and lead to breakouts known as **acne cosmetica**. Men need to learn about their skin type and how to prepare their skin properly for shaving. Everyone can learn the benefits of monthly or bi-monthly professional facials, regardless of how naturally smooth their complexions are.

The Thirties

In today's world, thirty is still a young age. Your clients may not be married yet, or if they are they may just be thinking about having children. In fact, this is often a prime age for personal services for those who are established in careers but not yet focused inward on their families. Roughly 35 to 45 percent of a typical business consists of clients who are between thirty and forty-five years old.

This is a critical age for starting to double up on skin protection, as this is the age when skin elasticity can start to "give" if one gets too much sun, drinks too much alcohol, smokes cigarettes, or skimps on sleep. This is the time to encourage clients to begin using eye cream and to use more sun protection products on a daily basis. It's also the age group with which to start discussing or publicizing special, targeted facial treatments. (**Fig. 1.3**)

Certain key age landmarks can appear during these years. For more and more women, these are the childbearing years,

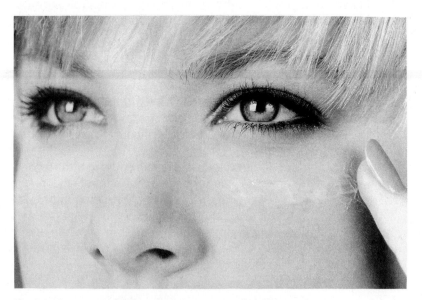

Fig. 1.3. Encourage the use of eye cream on a daily basis.

and pregnancy can change the texture of the skin, not just during pregnancy but afterwards. Hands may become drier than ever before; this is the first place subtle signs of aging often develop. Stress can start showing its effects on the body, especially if it's accompanied by inadequate exercise. Massage and other pampering treatments become increasingly appealing to this age group, so take the time to educate your clientele to the possibilities your salon offers.

The Forties

For many people today, the forties is the most exciting decade of their lives. They know who they are, they have tasted a bit of life's satisfaction, whether in their families or their careers, and they feel full of energy and enthusiasm.

Whereas forty was once seen as a demarcation of aging, today it is true that "life begins at forty." As mentioned earlier, it is also a key age group (especially forty to forty-five) for skin care salon clients. At this point, many clients come to you for the first time because they have started to see signs of aging despite the fact that they *feel* quite young. They trust that they can do something to keep their appearance as youthful as their spirits and energy, and they soak up information as fast as you can give it to them. This is a prime age group for salons that organize their offerings around educating their clients as much as treating them.

Skin tends to get drier and more fragile, and to show signs of stress faster, during the forties. Sunscreen is a must, as are moisturizers, eye creams, and monthly facials, especially in urban areas where pollution can make skin look tired even when a person is wide awake. Water-based foundations are important for women to help nourish the moisture needs of the skin. Alcohol-based toners should be abandoned, because they are too drying for most skin types at this point; water-based liquid makeup removers are a better bet for cleansing away foundation and dirt.

The Fifties

The fifties is the decade for reaping rewards—from friendships, family, work, hobbies—and for looking in the mirror and seeing the rewards of having taken care of one's skin (or, if one has been neglectful, of really seeing premature aging start to make itself known). At this point, the rule of thumb for skin maintenance is the gentler the better. No high heat, via steam, sauna, or heatlamps; no harsh products; no scrubbing or overzealous manipulation of skin. The less the skin is subjected to, the better. A basic cleansing routine, skin-kind makeup products, and richer, gentler facials and skin pampering treatments are the best choices.

For women, this can be an age of skin havoc, as **menopause** can make skin look old before its time. It may sap color from the skin, temporarily taking away its usual glow. The hot flashes that often accompany menopause can make makeup seem to melt into the skin, while water retention can make the face look puffy. Happily, once a woman goes through the process, there is often the nice surprise of looking like herself again. When **estrogen** is prescribed to help balance the body, it often helps the skin as well, as does taking recommended doses of vitamins including C and E (although E should never be used on facial skin, since it can clog the pores). It's a good idea to offer special attention to women clients if they complain that their skin doesn't have its usual color or elasticity anymore; simple adjustments of their skin care and makeup routines can often make a major difference in how they look and feel about themselves.

The Sixties and Beyond

At one time, one would never have expected to see many grandparents in a skin care salon; today, that has definitely changed. Just as people no longer consider sixty-five to be over the hill professionally or personally, so we need to recognize that older skin merits as much or more attention than younger skin. After all, persons who are still going to work, exercising, traveling, and volunteering for their favorite charities are not people whose appearance should be neglected. In fact, the soothing and pampering treatments that have been the hallmark of European skin care for decades are just the ticket for skin care during one's sixties and beyond.

It's not uncommon for clients in this age group to use a plastic surgeon's services. Skin care salons that recognize this can help to prepare for the "before" and "after" surgery stages (see chapter 9). In fact, more and more surgeons are seeking the advice estheticians can offer their patients to help smooth the transition back to an active life after the surgical healing period is complete.

This is also a time of important skin maintenance, when dryness or flakiness can escalate and important skin care choices may have to change. Offering free consultations for those celebrating landmark birthdays may bring in a surprising number of newly loyal clients for the effective pampering a skin care salon can provide.

SELF-QUIZ: QUESTIONS TO CONSIDER

Many of my clients claim that stress upsets their skin, but most textbooks claim that skin condition is a physical issue, not an emotional one. Which is correct?

Author's Advice: Although scientists still don't know the exact mechanisms, there is more and more agreement among top dermatologists that one's emotions are reflected in the skin. Acne, psoriasis, and eczema are all acknowledged to have emotional components; although they are actual physical conditions, they can be triggered or aggravated by stress. Similarly, rashes can sometimes flare up or subside depending on a person's emotional ups and downs.

One thing is certain: The pampering and relaxation that are part of skin care salon services are a very important part of the product that we deliver. That is why so much care should be taken in creating the right atmosphere, focusing on the client's needs, and never hurrying a facial or body treatment. It is also true that many of the most severe skin problems in which stress plays a role should be referred to a dermatologist, who can often work in conjunction with a skin care salon to provide a person with the best possible skin results.

I have recently moved to a big city from a more suburban area and am seeing more and more clients with Hispanic backgrounds. Many of them claim that their skin is oily, but it doesn't always seem that way. How common is dry skin among Hispanics?

Author's Advice: Many Hispanics, like many other Americans, are of mixed ethnic backgrounds today. Although it was once conventionally taught that Hispanic skin tends to be oily, it is very often combination skin, with areas that are dry (such as the cheeks and jaw area) and others that are oily (most often in the T-zone running across the forehead and down the nose). The best facial treatments, then, would utilize a mixture of oil-absorbing products to be used on oily areas and more nourishing, moisturizing products to be used on dryness-prone areas. The best at-home prescription would be to use normalizing cleansers that neither strip the skin too harshly nor are too creamy in consistency.

In general, it's important to trust your own instincts and educated examination of each client's skin rather than to over-rely on generalizations about various ethnic skin types. General guidelines are meant only as a starting point, not as a replacement for the reality you see when you examine a client's complexion under the magnifying light.

Anti-Aging and Skin Firming Techniques

The Ionic Facial Toning "Lift" as well as masks, ampoules, and injections help reduce the signs of aging and skin damage (Refer to Chapter 9, The Anti-Aging Game: What Skin Care Can Offer).

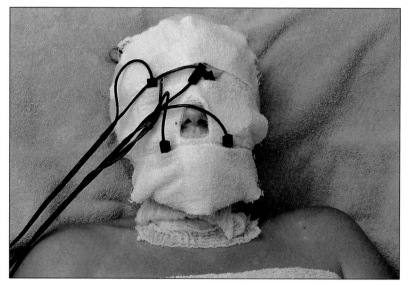

Plate 6: The electronic probe machine: probes are placed in gauze pockets.

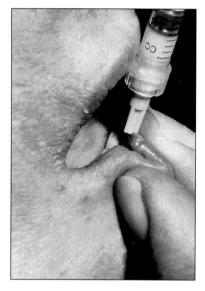

Plate 7: A filler injection

Skin Conditions

Skin conditions are often a result of overexposure to harsh weather and sun (Refer to Chapter 2, The Skin Exam).

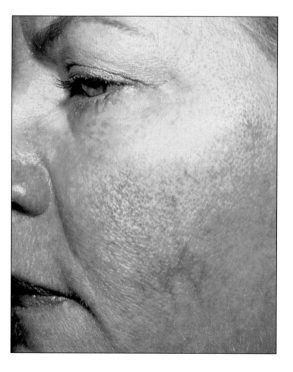

Plate 8: Broken capillaries. *Plate 8 courtesy of Dr. Timothy Berger.*

The chemical peel strips away all the layers of the epidermis and the very top of the dermis, leaving very red, very oozy skin that literally stimulates the growth of brand new skin (Refer to Chapter 9, The Anti-Aging Game: What Skin Care Can Offer).

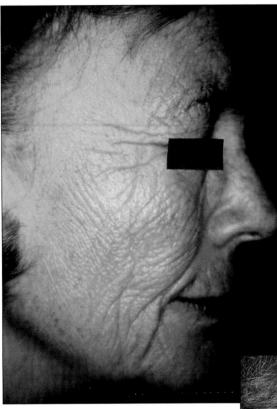

Plate 4: Before the chemical peel.

Plate 5: After the chemical peel. Surface lines disappear.

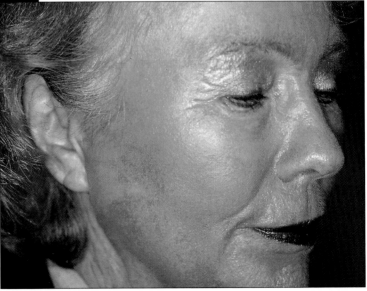

For clients whose skin really needs a lift, who have uneven pigmentation, fine lines, acne scars, and/or sun damage, there is the option of a salon deep peel (Refer to Chapter 9, The Anti-Aging Game: What Skin Care Can Offer).

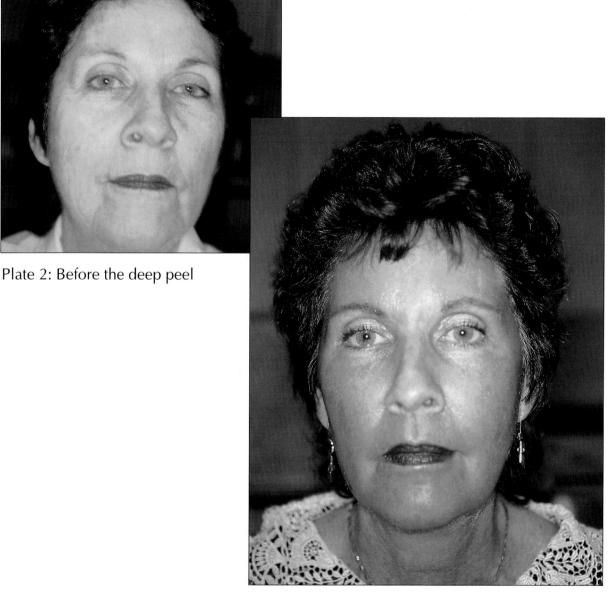

Plate 2: Before the deep peel

Plate 3: After the deep peel. The skin has improved tone, elasticity, texture, and color.

In an average square inch of skin, there are approximately 20 blood vessels, 65 hairs, 100 or more oil glands, 650 or more sweat glands, 28 nerves, 13 sense receptors for cold, 78 heat sensors, and 1,300 sensors to respond to touch (Refer to Chapter 1, Skin Basics: Understanding How the Skin Works).

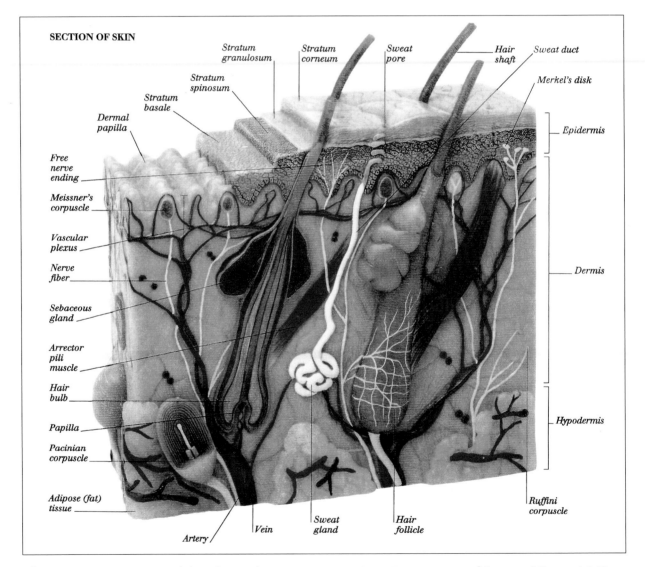

Plate 1: Cross section of the skin. *Plates 1, 2, 3, 4, 5, 6, 7 courtesy of Steven Victor, M.D.*

CHAPTER 2   The Skin Exam

In this chapter, you will learn how to perform the first, most important step of every facial: the skin exam. This includes:

- how to greet the client and put the client at ease,
- how to analyze the client's skin
- how to assess the impact of the client's lifestyle on the client's skin care needs.

In short, this chapter addresses everything that takes place before you actually give a client a skin treatment.

Your clients may think that skin treatment is the first or only thing that happens in a skin care salon, but a good esthetician knows that what takes place before the facial is actually the most important element of truly excellent skin care, because the skin exam is the basis for the proper choice of both salon and at-home services and products. It is also the first contact that most clients have with you as an esthetician and is your chance to make a good first impression that can translate into years of loyalty to your services.

MEETING AND GREETING: FIRST IMPRESSIONS

Before you even say hello to clients, you should know something about them. If the clients are regular customers of the salon, you will either know them (and their skin needs) personally, or you will have a folder that tells you their skin type and the type of facial they usually receive. If a client is new to the salon, that should be noted in the appointment book and you should be informed of it ahead of time. In either case, your role begins as soon as you say hello to the client.

It is important that you welcome every client to the salon and make each one feel comfortable in the treatment room. Your manner should be friendly and warm, caring but professional. It is customary at most salons to ask clients if they would like something to drink, such as spring water or herbal tea. The treatment room should be neat and scrupulously clean, with fresh towels, blankets, and robes prepared ahead of time for each client.

First-time clients require special attention to introduce them to the salon, as this is literally their first impression. Here are the best ways to introduce them to your salon and the skin care process.

- **Begin with a smile**. This may sound foolish or self-evident, but it is very important. Whether clients are getting their very first facials or are simply making their first visits to one particular salon, chances are they may feel a bit apprehensive. It is important that they be made to feel at ease. The best way to do that is for all salon personnel to be friendly and professional but not intimidating.

- **Give them a short tour of the salon**. If the receptionist or salon owner has not already done so, the esthetician should walk each client through the salon, briefly describing the services that are given in various areas. This serves three purposes. The client can be shown the cleanliness and professionalism of the entire salon in one quick step. She or he can also get a brief rundown of the variety of services offered. Whether the salon is very large or quite small, by the time you bring the client into the treatment room, it will feel like a familiar (not threatening) place. Then you, the esthetician, will be able to begin your examination of the client's skin without the client feeling that she or he is under a magnifying glass.

- **Invite the client to have a seat in the treatment room and explain that you (or the salon owner) would like to take a look at her or his skin**. You will, of course, have already observed some general parameters about the client's skin, such as whether it is overly dry or oily. In some salons, the next step is to ask the client to change into a robe, but this can be too much for a first-time client. Simply drape a clean towel over the client's shoulders, offer a headband to a woman if she would like to keep her hair off her face, and explain that you would like to cleanse off any makeup before you look at her skin.

TAKING A CLOSE LOOK: THE ART OF THE SKIN EXAM

The first step of the skin exam is to cleanse the skin surface of any makeup or dirt. Long hair should be held off the face with a terry cloth turban or headband. Jewelry and eyeglasses should be removed and placed in the client's purse or pocket, so they do not become coated with any products used. Ask if the client wears contact lenses; if so, they should be removed and put safely in a case before any skin treatment or exam is started. Then the skin should be cleansed, using the gentlest cleanser and toner available in the salon, so that you do not risk irritating the skin in any way.

It is then up to you to learn as much as possible about the client's skin. The first way to do this is by looking closely at the skin's surface.

- Look at the skin's overall color and texture. Does it look smooth and even, or are there blemishes or irritated areas? Do you see signs of aging or sun damage? Is there a healthy color to the skin? Are there any ashy patches, lines, or wrinkles? All of these questions provide clues to the overall vigor of the skin.

- Feel the skin's texture. Gently touch the skin using the thumb and index finger of one hand. Does it feel firm to the touch? As you press it in gently, does it spring back quickly? If you pull at it very, very gently, does it also spring back quickly? It's easiest to give this elasticity test while examining the skin under the magnifying light, because you can pull at the skin ever so gently and see the results magnified for you.

- Are there uneven, flaky patches that seem to lift up off the surface? Are there parched or red-looking areas? These are potential signals of dryness.

- Look at the skin on the nose and across the brows—the so-called **T-zone**. Is the skin shiny? Do you see oil on the surface? Are any blackheads or under-the-skin eruptions visible to the naked eye? If so, the skin in this area is oily, a condition that is common even when other areas of the face are dry. (**Fig. 2.1**)

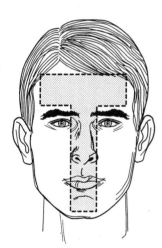

Fig. 2.1. The T-zone is often oily, even when other areas are dry.

Skin Characteristics

Now, it's time to take out the lighted skin magnifier. In most salons, this magnifying lens will be mounted on a swing-arm on the wall, making it easy to move it into place in front of the client. There are several important skin characteristics to look at.

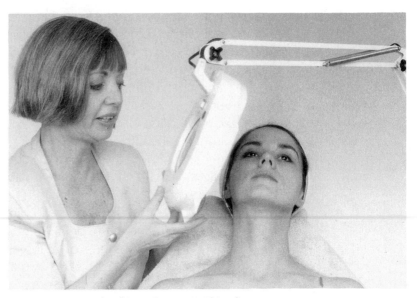

Fig. 2.2. Examine the skin under a magnifying lamp.

- Look for surface oil under the lamp. (**Fig. 2.2**) Do you see shiny areas? Examine the skin thoroughly from hairline to chin (two spots where you often see excess oil). Are there blackheads or skin eruptions around the hairline? If so, the client may be using hair products that are causing the problem.

- Examine the pores, especially on the nose. Are they empty and clear-looking? Is oil collected in them, giving them a blackened look under magnification? If the only pores that look clogged are on the nose, the client's skin may not be excessively oily. However, if you also see clogged pores on the cheeks and chin, then the skin is probably oily and also in need of a more thorough cleansing.

- Check for signs of sun damage. Do you see a network of tiny lines around the eyes? Does the skin look loose, especially around the eyes, mouth, or chin/neck areas? Feel the skin around the mouth. Does it feel firm and tight, or has it loosened? As people grow older, it is usual for the skin to "loosen" slightly (lose some elasticity), but take note if the degree of skin laxness seems greater than expected for a person of a given age.

- Finally, check for signs of skin sensitivity. Whether the skin is dry, oily, or combination, watch for red blotches, broken capillaries, fine spidery lines, and isolated flakiness.

DETERMINING SKIN TYPE: GETTING DOWN TO DETAILS

In most cases, of course, your clients will not have extreme problems but simply want to maintain or improve their skin's condition. Many skin experts emphasize the importance of knowing each person's skin type, dividing all skins precisely into categories of dry, oily, and combination. Because most salons today offer a wide variety of facials, it's also key to classify skin in terms of sun damage, texture, and sensitivity. In many cases, then, you can assign two or three skin types to one person's skin. Following are checklists of skin characteristics to help you confirm that your findings are accurate.

Oily Skin

1. **Extra shine**. Oily skin has an overall shiny look, even under makeup, and feels a bit greasy to the touch. In skin that is well cared for, this shininess need not be a negative; it can give skin the dewy look that many people like.

2. **A generally youthful appearance**. The one side benefit of excess skin oil is that skin does not wrinkle prematurely, but remains soft and pliable well into the forties, fifties, and often even sixties.

3. **The tendency to break out**. Oily skin types are more prone to skin eruptions, although they may not be severe and may only be in isolated areas. In a person who wears glasses, for example, you may observe clogged pores along the sides of the nose where the glasses rest. Blemishes might be concentrated under the chin, for example, in someone who talks on the phone a good deal or rests one hand under the chin while working or talking.

4. **Blackheads, especially on the nose and chin**. These may also occur along the hairline, as a result of sweat or the added pore-clogging effects of hair conditioners, sprays, mousses, or pomades.

5. **Whiteheads**. These pinhead-sized white bumps with no visible pore openings rarely occur on skins that are not excessively oily.

6. **Enlarged pores in general**. Even when skin is kept free of blemishes, pore openings will appear to be flatter and more open in an oily complexion, since at one time or another the pores will have held larger amounts of skin oils.

SPOTLIGHT

In my twenty-five years in the skin care business, I've found that most people have the wrong assumptions about their skin. I remember one instance very clearly. When I first interviewed a new client in my salon, she told me that her skin was oily. To my eye, her skin looked extremely sensitive; upon closer examination, I noticed how dry and flaky her skin was, although it had the most beautiful elasticity. What was most obvious to me, in fact, was that I couldn't notice any surface oil at all.

I questioned this young woman further and found that, because she had a few blackheads, she assumed her skin was oily and needed vigorous cleansing. Her skin care regimen, she told me, consisted of soap and plain rubbing alcohol; she was afraid to use a moisturizer, she said, because of her blackheads and oily skin. I explained the condition of her skin to her and recommended that she use cleansing lotion instead of soap, along with a light moisturizer to protect her skin. A peeling mask to slough off the dead cells, I told her, would also help; the cleansing of regular facials would easily remove the few blackheads she had.

This young woman wasn't at all receptive at first, but I persuaded her to give it a chance and she did. Two weeks later, she came back into the salon with a huge smile and said, "You were right. I will always listen to your advice."

Dry Skin

1. **A matte finish**. Before and after cleansing, skin looks flat and doesn't reflect very much light.

2. **Oversensitivity to cold weather**. In wintertime, dry skin will always look a bit parched and, in a Caucasian person, slightly reddish in tone.

3. **Minimal perspiration**, regardless of the temperature.

4. **Rough, flaky areas**. These may only appear after cleansing, since moisturizer can keep these in check.

5. **Fine lines and wrinkles on a person in the thirties**. Although premature aging may not be severe if a person has used adequate sun protection, in general, dry-skinned individuals age sooner than those with oily complexions.

Combination Skin

1. **An oily T-zone**, which encompasses the forehead, nose, and chin. This area may simply be excessively shiny, or may suffer from breakouts on or below the skin surface.

2. **Oily or pimpled hairline**.

3. **Smooth or just slightly dry cheeks**. They may have isolated dry patches, or in some cases, cheeks may even be so dehydrated that they are very flaky.

4. **Clogged pores on the nose or chin**.

5. **Dryness under the eyes or around the upper lip**. In some people, this is the only area that becomes dry and flaky.

Acne-Prone Skin

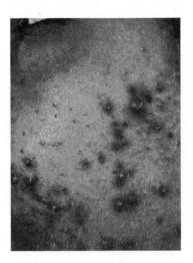

Fig. 2.3. Acne. (Courtesy of Timothy Berger, M.D.)

1. **Oiliness** that results in skin looking shiny regardless of the time of day. Skin usually looks oily even under makeup.

2. **Very enlarged, clogged pores**, not just on the nose but around the edges of the face—hairline and chin especially.

3. **Breakouts**. These may be blackheads or whiteheads.

4. **Raised comedones**, closed pimples underneath the skin surface. (**Fig. 2.3**)

5. **Scars from picking at the skin**. Many people whose skin has a tendency toward eruptions will pick at blemishes in an effort to speed their clearing. Of course, the opposite occurs: Skin that is picked at becomes more inflamed, infected, and aggravated. The end result is often a **depressed scar**, a flat area of hard skin that is very difficult to clear up. Ironically, some of the people who pick at their skin the most actually have the least severe breakouts; it is the sight of a single pimple on an otherwise clear complexion that sends them into a frenzy.

Sun-Damaged Skin

1. **Fine lines around the eyes**. These may be due to squinting or actual direct exposure to ultraviolet light.

2. **Wrinkling around the mouth**. The lip area has little natural protection against the sun, so it is often one of the first places to show sun-induced wrinkling.

3. **"Loose" skin at a young age**. Because sun exposure breaks down the skin's supportive network of collagen and elastin, those who get too much sun will have lax skin around the mouth and chin or neck area at a younger age than should be expected.

4. **Leathery texture**. On touching the skin, it may feel rough and hardened rather than soft and smooth. Or it may seem very fragile (see item 5 in this list).

5.   **Thin, fragile-feeling texture**. In people with very fair complexions, the sun's ultraviolet light may cause skin to thin out, with the result that it feels—and is—fragile to the touch.

6.   **Dark spots**. Often called age or liver spots, these are most often seen on the hands but may also show up on the face. (**Fig. 2.4**)

Sensitive Skin

1.   **Thin skin**. An inherited trait most often found in redheads and blonds (though not exclusive to the fair haired). It almost always means perpetual sensitivity.

2.   **Broken capillaries**. More precisely, this condition of thread-like, spidery red lines around the nose or cheeks is due to lack of capillary elasticity, which results in capillaries that, after

SPOTLIGHT
••••••••••••••••••

As a skin care professional, I've learned that how you tell clients something is as important as what you tell them. For example, some clients are always surprised that I can tell that they pick on their skin. "How did you know?" they ask, when the results are obviously written on their faces. The first client whose skin revealed this to me also taught me an important lesson: a smile can go a long way in any communication.

The thirty-year-old woman was a first-time visitor to my salon, although she told me she had had "a lot of facials, on and off, in different salons." "And you have also been trying to clean out some breakouts on your own at home, I see," I said to her with a great big smile on my face—more out of embarrassment at what I heard myself saying than out of amusement, I admit. She reacted by admitting that yes, she had. "How did you know?" she asked, incredulously. "I'm a skin care expert with knowledge and experience," I responded. "I'm supposed to know." After that, the ice was broken between us and I was able to talk to her about the need to be gentle with her skin—and to plead with her not to pick at her skin anymore. I explained that by picking, she was simply spreading the infection and fighting a never-ending battle; by stopping, she could clear up her skin in a matter of weeks.

I didn't know if my speech had had any effect until four weeks later, when she called to make an appointment for another facial. "My skin really looks better," she told me. "I'm not picking at it anymore. And thanks," she added, "for not lecturing at me like my mom."

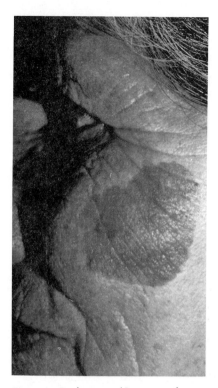

Fig. 2.4. Dark spots. (Courtesy of Timothy Berger, M.D.)

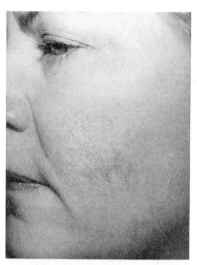

Fig. 2.5. Broken capillaries. (Courtesy of Steve Victor, M.D.)

they expand from blushing, cold, or heat, don't contract totally but remain overexpanded. Other causes include too much sun exposure, excessive alcohol intake, or rough handling of delicate skin. (**Fig. 2.5**)

3. **Blotchiness on otherwise smooth skin**. A complexion that is sensitive is often uneven in coloration, as one area of the face may react when another skin area doesn't. This is especially true in women, because some sensitivity is due to makeup ingredients. The makeup that a woman uses on one part of the face only may be at fault.

4. **Hives**. These may or may not be present when you examine someone's skin, but if they are, it's often sensitivity rather than a true allergic reaction. The culprit is often a skin care ingredient, either something used on the face or, often, on the hands and transferred to facial skin when a person touches the face.

5. **Itching and flaking**. This is often the result of temperature extremes, whether heat or cold, or anything that brings a flush to the face, such as spicy foods, saunas, or steam rooms. It can also result from overly harsh cleansing, whether in product choice or overuse of a washcloth.

NOTE: Every person's skin is sensitive to some degree; just about everyone may react to something in the environment at

some time or another. But some complexions are especially vulnerable to irritation, whether from chemicals, makeup ingredients, or environmental factors from wind to pollution. The traits
described here apply to those skin types that are most highly
sensitive; those who have sensitive skin may have all, some, or
just one of these characteristics.

TAKE A SKIN HISTORY

Looking at the skin isn't the only way to determine its condition.
You will also want to ask the client some questions, either
while you examine the skin or, preferably, right afterward. Most
people, even those who have beautiful complexions and come
for regular facials, often think that they have problem skin.
Part of the esthetician's job is to be encouraging about each
client's complexion, so that they will take pleasure in caring for
themselves. There are several ways to approach this subject:

- **Start with positive feedback**. The most common time for
  clients to feel apprehensive is when you have turned the
  magnifying light onto their skin; after all, no one feels so confident in their appearance that they feel they can look great
  under such conditions. For that reason, this is the best
  time to find something positive to say about the skin, to help
  put the client at ease. (**Fig. 2.6**) If a woman's skin has a
  wonderful peaches-and-cream tone, you might say, "Your skin

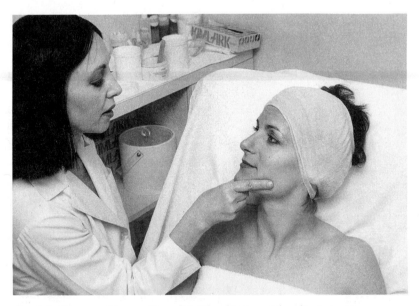

Fig. 2.6. Say something positive about the skin to put the client at ease.

has a very healthy color," for example; if a man's beard has been nicely trimmed and his skin doesn't exhibit any razor irritation, you might note, "Your complexion has a nice smooth texture."

These types of positive comments are especially important in cases in which you do see problems in someone's complexion, such as a tendency to blemishes or premature sun damage. The chances are that the woman or man who has come to you with a skin problem is hoping that you will help solve it. The first, most crucial step you can take is to give the client a positive feeling about having come to you for your expertise.

- **Ask every client the basic three: work, home, and habits**. The three factors that are most likely to have an effect on people's skin, either right now or in the future, are their job, where they live, and how they take care of their skin.

  You must ask about these three factors, however, with a certain degree of delicacy. Some clients may choose to tell their skin care advisors (like their hairdressers) many details of their private lives, but it is not a skin care advisor's place to pry. Instead, it is wise to preface your questions with a comment such as, "I'd like to ask you a few questions that can help me to help you to take better care of your skin, since we find that people's lifestyles can have a big impact on their complexions." Because not everyone who comes to a salon works outside the home, for example, you might ask "Do you work outside the home?" rather than "What is your profession?" The reason you want to know this is that on-the-job stress is a frequent contributor to many skin problems, as are frequent travel, climate changes, and the harsh chemicals that are a factor in many professions. A man with oily skin, for example, who works in an overheated dry cleaning store may need more frequent or more intensive skin treatments than someone who works in an air-conditioned office or outside on a construction site.

  Learning where a person lives is important because of the many negative effects that pollution can have on skin, contributing to clogged pores and breakouts. A client who lives in one climate during the winter months and another during the summer months will also have differing skin needs in the future than someone who lives in the same city year-round.

Perhaps the most crucial question of all to ask is what kind of skin care routines clients follow right now. What types of cleansing products do they use? How often? Any astringents, toners, or home masks? Are they under a dermatologist's care? Do they use any prescription products on their skin?

- **Check for any medical factors right away**. Before you give anyone a facial, you should always be sure to ask whether they are under any type of medical treatment that would make them sensitive to anything you might use. There are four things that every esthetician should ask each new client:

    1. Do you have a heart condition? (Care must often be taken to avoid extreme heat, even such as steaming; a pacemaker makes the use of certain facial machines unwise.)

    2. Do you have diabetes? (If the answer is yes, you should ask if they have any circulation disorders that would make the use of steaming or massage a problem.)

    3. (If the client is a woman) Are you pregnant? (It is best to avoid use of all machines in this case, since there may be unknown dangers.)

    4. Are you using **retinoic acid,** commonly known as **Retin-A**?* (If so, the skin will be extremely sensitive and all but the gentlest facials then become out of the question.)

    As with all questions that you ask your clients, these should be presented in a soft-spoken, professional manner, not in an alarmist or intimidating way. The idea is to let the client know that you want to be sure you have important information, not that you are giving him or her the third degree. One way to make this easier for both you and the client is to interject a comment at some point such as, "I'm sorry to ask so many personal questions, but it will help me to take better care of your skin."

- **If you see a skin problem, ask, kindly, for more detail**. To help clients who have blemishes or very, very dry skin, you will need a bit more information about their lives. But you want to be especially sensitive in asking further questions,

---

* Though there are other manufacturers of retinoic acid, this text will refer specifically to Retin-A™—not as an endorsement, but because it is the commonly recognized term used in the industry.

because a client with problem skin is probably a bit emotionally sensitive about the subject as well. On the average, for every fifteen to twenty people who visit a skin care salon, there are four or five who do have problem skin, whether it's excessive oiliness and random breakouts or excessive irritation and flakiness. In this case, it makes sense to ask about factors that can affect the skin, such as whether the person is under stress; if she travels a good deal (for example, a flight attendant may have developed extremely dry skin from the dehydrating effects of plane travel); if she exercises (if a woman has breakouts, it's sometimes due to not removing makeup thoroughly beforehand); if he uses saunas (another potential oil promoter); or if there's anything in the client's life right now that she or he thinks may be affecting the skin. Try to listen as much as or more than you probe. Clients often have concerns that they want to talk about that may be tangential to what you are asking, but are important to pay attention to; a salon visit should involve an exchange of information. One caveat: Don't expect—or even try—to get all the information you need on the first visit.

- **Be on the lookout for people who should not have facials**. Part of being a responsible esthetician is realizing that some skin conditions require medical attention, such as severe **cystic acne** or **eczema**. Although facials can do a great deal to clear up blemishes, those that are severely infected or inflamed require a dermatologist's attention first. You should delicately inform anyone who has cystic acne and comes to your salon seeking a facial that it could actually make the condition worse rather than better, that she or he should seek a dermatologist's care first and then come back to help keep the skin clear (in fact, many salons regularly work with specific dermatologists in a treatment partnership of this type). Similarly, you should not attempt to give a facial to anyone who has severe eczema in which the skin is irritated to the point of bleeding or cracking.

  During the summer months, or during midwinter peak vacation seasons, you may also encounter some clients who come to the salon after getting a pretty severe sunburn. Because the steaming and massage of a facial could potentially increase the skin's irritation, it's also a good general rule to advise them to allow the skin time to recover first, then come back for a facial. You might recommend an aloe-vera-based cream or lotion to help speed the skin's self-healing process.

SELF-QUIZ: QUESTIONS TO CONSIDER

I am a pretty shy person. How can I ask someone so many questions about their skin?

Author's Advice: Gaining confidence in your own abilities as an esthetician is essential to being able to ask questions. For this reason, most reputable salons require that all new employees spend at least two weeks as apprentices or assistants, working with an experienced esthetician. As you spend time with clients day in and day out, you will see that striking up a conversation becomes easier. After all, most clients who come to a skin care salon come seeking advice and information. Because the questions you ask of them will help you to provide the most information possible, carrying on the dialogue will become a natural part of your job. If you feel truly intimidated about asking questions, try practicing with friends or family members.

I notice that you recommend examining first-time clients' skin while they still have their street clothes on. In many salons, the practice is for the receptionist to escort clients to the facial room and ask them to put on a robe before the esthetician arrives. Why don't you recommend this?

Author's Advice: Aside from allowing clients who are nervous about getting a first facial to stay a bit more relaxed, doing a skin exam while the client is still in street clothes allows the esthetician to analyze the client's overall image. The clothes that clients are wearing, their accessories, whether they wear glasses, how much makeup or jewelry they wear all become clues to help you determine the type of facial you will recommend, the type of skin care regimen you might advise, the frequency of visits, and the way in which your clients perceive themselves. For example, if you think that a woman's skin problem is due in part to her makeup, yet you have observed that she likes to wear a lot of makeup, then you realize you can't simply say, "Don't wear makeup." You will have to help her find products that achieve the look she's after without irritating her skin. In my experience, the practice of skin care is a combination of expert advice and armchair psychologist: You need to deliver advice in a way that makes sense to each individual's life. Seeing how they present themselves on an everyday basis, rather than having them change into robes before you even see them, helps you to know them a bit better. My recommendation may be a little less time-efficient, but I think it helps a salon provide the best service possible.

Is there a simple test that clients can do to analyze their skin at home? I find they often like to check on its progress.

Author's Advice: I often recommend the following cotton-ball test for use at home. Mix up this tonic: In a blender, combine the juice of one lemon, 1/2 cup distilled water, 1 teaspoon olive oil, and three ice cubes. Blend till the ice is melted. Then brush the hair off the face and cleanse the skin, using a gentle cleansing lotion. Finish by recleansing the skin using cotton balls wetted with the tonic. Wait three hours. Wet three cotton balls with the tonic. Using a circular motion, gently wipe the first cotton ball across the forehead, the second down the nose, and the third across one cheek. If all three come up clean, the skin is probably dry; if they're dark, it's oily; if they're slightly soiled, it's probably a combination of the two.

CHAPTER 3 The Basic Facial

In this chapter, you will learn how to give a complete, step-by-step facial designed to cleanse, smooth, and improve the skin. A high-quality, thorough facial features steps designed not only to nourish and care for the skin, but also to pamper the client. You will learn how to:

- organize the treatment room ahead of time to maximize the client's comfort and your own efficiency
- gently prepare the skin
- deliver a luxurious massage to the face and upper body (one of the most distinctive but too often overlooked steps of a truly great facial)
- completely clean out pores without damaging or marking the skin
- select and apply masks
- provide the relaxing finishing touch of a shoulder and hand massage.

All of the information in this chapter is aimed at the dual goals of providing the best possible cleansing and nourishing of the client's skin while at the same time providing a totally relaxing, pampering experience. Although some facialists are very good technicians, adept at cleansing the skin, and others are very good at making their clients feel cared for, the best possible facial treatment should combine the best of both worlds, leaving the client's skin looking and feeling better and the client feeling relaxed and pampered.

THE FACIAL ROOM: AN OASIS OF PEACE

Before a proper facial can be given, the treatment room must be set up properly. At the start of each day, adequate supplies should be on hand in each room. These supplies include cleansers, toners, cotton, creams, masks, and the all-important spatulas to be used to remove all creams, cleansers, and

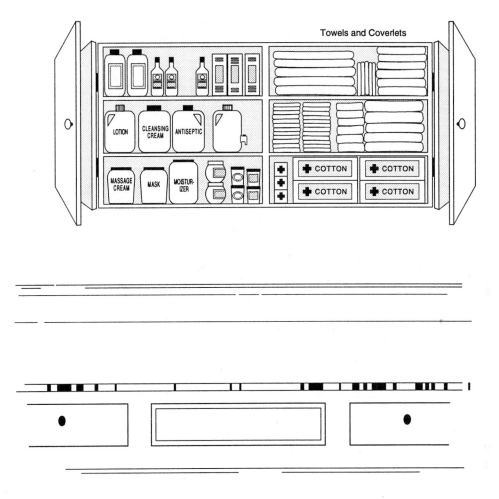

Fig. 3.1. A facial room should be clean, organized, and well stocked.

masks from their containers (fingers should *never* be used to dip into containers). Your supplies should be organized in a closed cabinet if at all possible; if they must be kept on a small tabletop, all containers should be closed to avoid the dustiness and contamination that can develop almost instantly. Extra jars and rolls of sterile absorbent cotton should be kept in a cabinet in the room, immediately available so that you do not run out of something in the middle of a facial. It should never be necessary for a facialist to leave the room in search of additional moisturizer or whatever. (**Fig. 3.1**)

Before the client is brought into the room, the chair should be covered with a clean sheet and fresh towels. Depending on the time of year and the temperature in the salon, there should be blankets or oversize towels to cover the client if she or he wishes. A clean robe should be provided for each client, and a towel or headband should be given to anyone who wants to further protect the hair from contact with creams and masks.

Each client should be given absolute privacy to change into a robe and get settled in the treatment chair. Then the esthetician should come back into the room and the lights should be dimmed to a relaxing level. You should then wash your hands in the presence of the client, announcing "I'm going to wash my hands now" as a routine way of providing the reassurance that your hands are as clean as all the other equipment in the salon. Always ask if the client is comfortable—warm or cool enough, if the chair is comfortable or needs to be adjusted.

CLEANSING: HOW TO PREPARE THE SKIN FOR TREATMENT

Many clients come to a salon in the middle of a work day, or even at the end of one, so their skin requires a gentle but complete surface cleansing to prepare it for the benefits of a facial. Because the majority of those who come for facials are women, this section describes the cleansing assuming that the client is wearing makeup; in the case of a woman who isn't wearing any makeup, or when the client is a man, simply omit the makeup-removing steps.

Eye makeup should always be removed before any other cleansing is done to avoid accidentally smudging any of it into a client's eyes (and, of course, contact lenses should be removed beforehand). Because the eye area is so sensitive, it is always a good idea to ask a new client, or one whom you have not treated before, whether she has any allergies to cleansers before beginning. In general, using a liquid makeup remover is the best choice for cleansing away all mascara and shadow. A liquid doesn't spread or burn the eyes, is least likely to cause eye irritation, and is quicker to use than a cream or gel. The speed with which an eye-makeup remover works is key to its gentleness: the less rubbing that is needed, the less likely the eyes are to become red or teary. What you use to apply the makeup remover (and all cleansers) to the skin is also crucial. Sterile absorbent cotton that comes in a roll is a much better choice than cotton balls, because it is the softest grade of cotton available and can be customized in size for your cleansing needs. It's

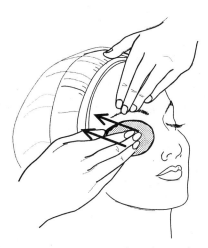

Fig. 3.2. Apply cotton from the inside of eye to the outside.

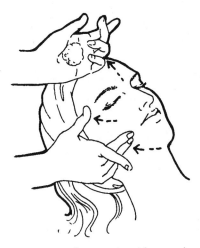

Fig. 3.3. Work cream in with a gentle upward motion.

best to use pieces of cotton that are about two inches square; that way, you can fold it up to a smaller size and keep opening it up and refolding it several times until you have used all of the surfaces.

To apply liquid eye-makeup remover, saturate a piece of cotton and then squeeze it out. Use a gentle motion moving from the inside of the eye to the outside. (**Fig. 3.2**) Repeat, gently, until all eye makeup is removed (you may want to use a cotton swab to clean up any stray liner or mascara). Follow by repeating the same motion with cotton simply dipped in cool water. This will cool and soothe the eye area.

NOTE: You can never be too gentle when cleansing the skin, but this is especially true when working around the eyes, the most delicate area of all.

Next, use a creamy cleanser, again applied with cotton squares, all over the face. Most salons should have two types of cleansing cream, one that's lightweight, for normal to oily skin, and one that is richer, for extremely dry, fragile, or aging skin. Always apply the cleansing cream from the bottom of the face up, using a gentle motion, working against gravity to avoid stretching the skin. (**Fig. 3.3**) Although many facialists use sponges in cleansing, unless they are thrown away after each use (an extremely expensive, and thus impractical, idea), they're not a very good choice, as they can too easily become contaminated with bacteria. Never use tissue to cleanse the skin, except for the mouth. To remove lipstick, first use a tissue to blot it off, then follow with wet cotton and a creamy cleanser. Don't forget to cleanse the neck as well, working gently from the center outward. As a finishing step, take a piece of dry cotton and gently go over the skin with a toner (for dry skin), astringent (for oily skin), or cleansing lotion (for combination skin).

One way to evaluate whether you have given a client thorough preparation for the facial ahead is to look at the skin under the magnifying lamp at this point and be sure that it is bare of all makeup, oil, and dirt. Another is simply to glance at your watch: a good surface cleansing should take about five minutes. If you have finished taking off a woman's makeup in one minute, you probably haven't done as complete a job as you should have.

MASSAGE: THE ULTIMATE IN RELAXATION

What comes next can be considered the most important part of any facial. After all, if clients have pretty good skin, they may not feel that cleansing, even the pore cleansing that comes later in the facial, is that big a deal—but no one can match the pampering and relaxing effect of a great facial massage on their own at home. This is the part of a facial, you will find, that really keeps clients coming back for more. Also, the effect of that relaxation is often what helps the skin take on a healthy-looking glow. A good massage stimulates the skin to receive the benefits of masks and creams to be applied later; it increases circulation to the skin, at least temporarily; and it helps soften and smooth the skin's texture.

Before focusing on the precise technique, be sure you are in shape to give a good massage:

- Your nails should be short and rounded; if you're dedicated to having long nails, then you'll never be able to give a proper massage—and may risk stabbing a client as well!

- A facialist should never wear rings. Not only can they get covered with creams, but they could also be felt on the skin during a massage. (**Fig. 3.4**)

- Your hands should be flexible and relaxed but strong and confident. This is as much a reflection of how you feel about giving the massage as it is of how much experience and practice you get. The more you practice giving massages, the stronger your hands will become at it.

- Before beginning each massage, wash your hands in warm water and prepare a small bowl of warm water that you can dip into from time to time to be sure that your hands don't get

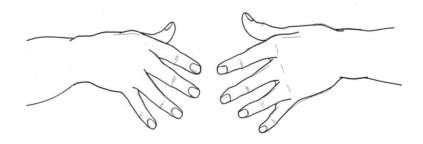

Fig. 3.4. A facialist should have short, rounded nails and avoid wearing rings and noisy jewelry.

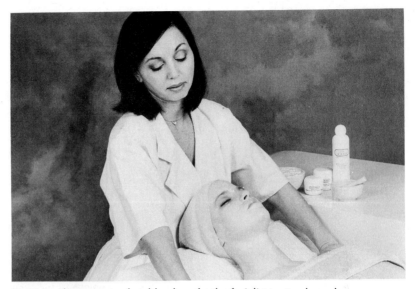

Fig. 3.5. The most comfortable place for the facialist to stand may be behind the client's chair.

cold. Not only is it harder to give a massage with cold hands, but it doesn't feel very good to the client.

You should also have an open container of massage cream nearby. Begin by smoothing some onto your hands—then you're ready to start the facial massage.

The method outlined here combines elements of European (or Swedish) and Eastern-inspired pressure-point massage techniques, for both stimulating and relaxing effects. It focuses on key areas—the temples, brows, and jaw—where many people store up tension in their faces. Throughout the massage, your fingers should be slightly curved, with just the fingertips touching the client's skin. Your hands should be loose, with the wrists and fingers flexible, so that you can conform your fingers to the shape of each area of the face. Because many of the movements involve working on each side of the client's face with both hands, one of the most comfortable places for you to stand may be behind the client's chair; other movements may be more easily performed while standing or sitting on one side of the client. (**Fig. 3.5**) Don't be concerned about getting each step of the massage precisely correct the first time you do it; what is crucial is that all your movements have a softness and fluidity to them. As you practice the massage, each step will become easier, more natural, and more fluid.

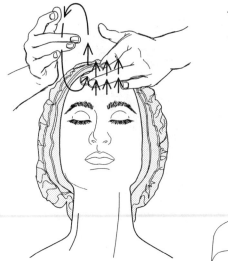

Fig. 3.6. Make linear movements over the forehead.

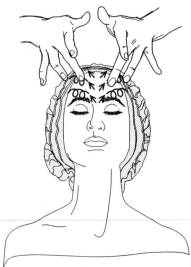

Fig. 3.7. Make circular movements on the forehead.

Procedures

1.   With the middle and ring fingers of each hand, start with gentle upward strokes in the middle of the forehead, working up from the browline to the hairline. Going along the hairline, move toward the right, with one hand following the other to the right temple. Continue the same movement working back across the forehead to the left temple. Then work back to the center of the forehead. Repeat several times. (**Fig. 3.6**)

2.   Using the middle fingers of each hand, start making small circular movements in the middle of the forehead between the brows. Continue these circular movements, moving the right hand toward the right temple and the left hand toward the left temple. As you reach the temples, bring the fingers back quickly to the center again and repeat the movements. After the second time, apply slight pressure to the temples and the brows before returning to the center. Repeat several more times, increasing the pressure at the temples ever so gently. (**Fig. 3.7**)

3.   Using the middle and ring fingers of each hand, place one hand above the other at the middle of the forehead. Then use a "crisscross" movement—alternating strokes with each hand—to move upward from the browline to the

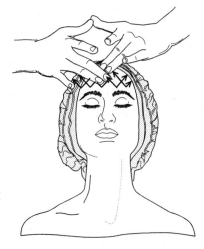

Fig. 3.8. The criss-cross movement.

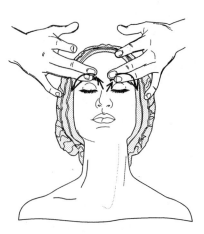

Fig. 3.9. Slightly lift the brows.

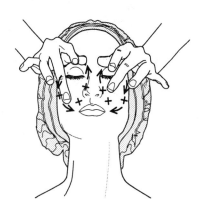

Fig. 3.10. Tap fingertips around the eyes.

hairline. Move toward the right temple and then back to the center; then move toward the left temple and back to the center. Repeat several times. (**Fig. 3.8**)

4. Place the ring fingers under the inside of each eyebrow and the middle fingers over each brow. Gently slide fingers to the outer corner of the eye, lifting the brows slightly at the same time. Then start making small circles with the middle finger at the outside corner of the eye. Continue these circular motions on the cheekbones underneath each eye (be sure you're on the bone, not on the fat pads underneath the eyes). Then slide fingers around the eyes back to the starting point. Repeat six to eight times. (**Fig. 3.9**)

5. Using the pads of your fingertips of each whole hand, lightly tap your fingers around each eye. Continuing this gentle tapping action, move out to the temples, then under the eyes toward the nose, then up and over the brows and back to the temples. Staying away from the eyelids, repeat this tapping circle six times. (**Fig. 3.10**)

6. With the middle fingers of each hand, start a gentle circular massage down the nose and continuing across each cheek to the temples. Slide the fingers under the eyes and back to the bridge of the nose. Repeat this "sinus movement" six times. (**Fig. 3.11**)

7. Using the middle and ring fingers of each hand, slide your fingers from the bridge of the nose over the brows and

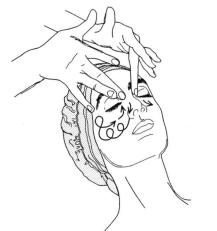

Fig. 3.11. Stimulate the sinus.

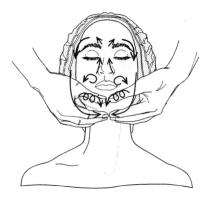

Fig. 3.12. Nose, brow, and chin movements.

down to the chin. Using your thumbs, start a firm circular motion on the chin, working from beneath the ears to the center of the jaw. Switch back to the middle fingers at the corners of the mouth, rotating your fingers there several times, then sliding your fingers up the sides of the nose, over the brows, and out to the temples. Stop at the temples for a moment, then slide fingers down to the chin and repeat the whole sequence several times. (**Fig. 3.12**)

8. With the middle finger of each hand, start a circular motion at the center of the chin and move out to each earlobe. Return fingers to the corners of the mouth, then continue movements out toward the middle of each ear. Using the same circular motion, work up along the edge of the face to a spot even with the top of each ear. Repeat several times. (**Fig. 3.13**)

9. Using the index and middle fingers of each hand, start a scissor-like movement above the center of the mouth, moving outward with each hand and up toward the cheekbones. Stop at the top of the cheekbones. Then return fingers to a point above the mouth, and repeat with right hand only, then with left hand only, alternating each side of the face. Repeat ten times. (**Fig. 3.14**)

10. Place the middle finger of each hand above the mouth. Gently slide fingers to outer corners of mouth, then under the lower lip down to the chin. Repeat eight times. (**Fig. 3.15**)

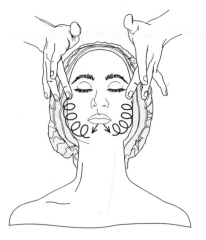

Fig. 3.13. Circulate from chin to earlobe.

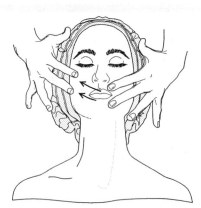

Fig. 3.14. Make a scissor-like movement around the mouth.

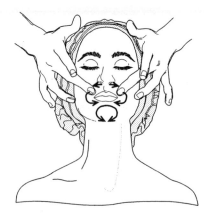

Fig. 3.15. Stimulate the chin and mouth.

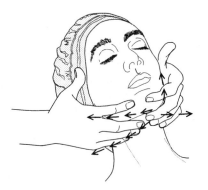

Fig. 3.16. Make a scissor-like movement around the jawline.

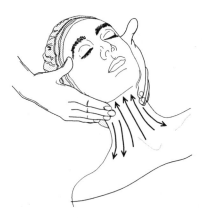

Fig. 3.17. Stroke the neck.

11. With the index fingers above the jawline and the middle fingers below, start a scissor action moving outward from the center of the chin toward the earlobes. Alternate hand movements, repeating ten times on each side of face. (**Fig. 3.16**)

12. Using four fingers of each hand, apply upward strokes over the front of the neck. Then use a firmer downward stroke on the sides of the neck in an oval-shaped motion. Repeat ten times. (**Fig. 3.17**)

13. With the middle and ring fingers of your right hand, give two fast taps under the chin on the far right side. Then follow with one tap from the middle and ring fingers of the left hand. Continue this rhythm, moving from right to left to cover the whole underside of the chin without stopping. (**Fig. 3.18**)

14. Continue the same tapping rhythm, this time starting on the right cheek and giving the left-hand single tap a slight lifting motion. Repeat this ten times without stopping, then switch to the left cheek and repeat ten times without stopping. (**Fig. 3.19**)

15. Without stopping the tapping motion, move back under the chin and over to just below the right corner of the mouth. Then switch to a circular or rolling motion with the first three fingers of each hand, one hand following the other as each finger lifts the right corner of the mouth. Repeat twenty times. Then switch to the left side and repeat twenty times. (**Fig. 3.20**)

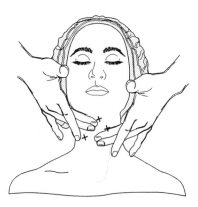

Fig. 3.18. Tap fingertips under the chin.

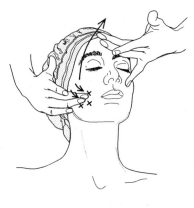

Fig. 3.19. Tap the cheeks.

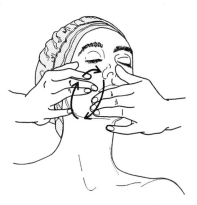

Fig. 3.20. Roll fingers around the mouth.

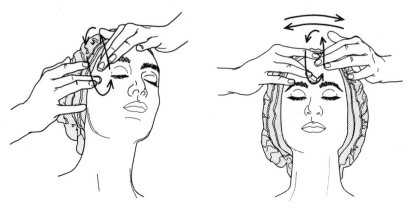

Fig. 3.21. Roll fingers around the eyes.

Fig. 3.22. Roll fingers across the forehead.

16. Continue the gentle rolling motion, using the first three fingers of each hand, and move up to the outer corners of the eyes. First, using the left hand, do twenty circles at the outer corner of the left eye. Then do twenty more at the outer corner of the right eye. **(Fig. 3.21)**

17. Using both hands, continue the gentle rolling movement back and forth across the forehead. Let the movements grow lighter and lighter until the fingers are gradually lifted from the forehead, after approximately ten to twenty sweeps across the forehead. **(Fig. 3.22)**

THE DREAM STEAMING: WARM AND WONDERFUL

The next step is the steaming, which softens the skin and helps prepare the pores for being thoroughly cleaned out. It is best to leave the skin as is after the massage; this way, the light coating of massage cream will protect the skin during the steaming process. Even if the client's skin is oily, leaving the massage cream on will help avoid any redness or broken capillaries.

Before starting the steaming, cover the client's shoulders, neck, and chest with a clean towel or sheet and *always* cover the client's eyes with cotton pads dipped in cool (but not too cold) water or in a **chamomile-based** eye wash. Place the steam machine approximately fifteen inches away from the face. **(Fig. 3.23)** Wait a few seconds to let the steam hit the face and then ask if the client is comfortable. Because different people have different thresholds for heat tolerance—and you can never

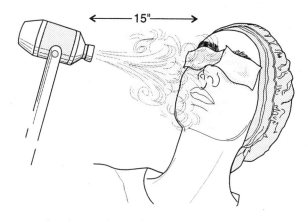

Fig. 3.23. Drape the client with towels and cover the eyes with cotton. The steamer should be approximately fifteen inches from the face.

be too sure that the machine is at the right setting—never run out of the room as soon as you set up the steam machine. Once you are certain that the client is comfortable, you can leave the room for a few minutes; always announce that you are leaving first, though. Don't leave for more than five minutes at the absolute most, since the maximum steaming time should be five to seven minutes. Pregnant women, of course, should never be left for that long; the maximum time to steam a pregnant woman's skin should be two minutes, because heat tolerance is reduced during pregnancy. If a client indicates that steaming isn't the favorite part of the facial, you can come back into the room sooner and ask if she'd like to stop the steam at that point.

In some salons, steam machines are not used; instead, boiling water is placed in a heat-resistant bowl, mixed with chamomile water, and then positioned where a gentle steam will reach the client. If you use this method, you must be especially careful that the bowl is sturdy and in a stable position.

At the end of the steaming, remove the eye compresses and go over the skin with cotton dipped in warm water and creamy cleanser to remove any perspiration or leftover massage cream.

PORE CLEANSING: THE WHOLE STORY

Cleaning out the pores is one of the most crucial—and most delicate—steps of a facial. It is the most thorough way to remove skin impurities, yet it needs to be done with the utmost care. Too rough pore cleansing will leave a client's skin red and irritated; too little cleansing of the pores, however, can result in skin that still looks a bit clogged after a facial.

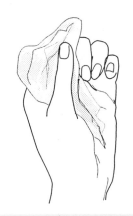

Fig. 3.24. The pore cleansing tool: secure a tissue around both index fingers.

Always put a fresh set of cool compresses over the client's eyes before beginning the cleansing process, as you will be putting on the bright magnifying light and you don't want to shine this light into the client's eyes. Take a tissue in your hands and fold it three times; put your two index fingers inside the tissue. This will be your pore-cleansing tool. (**Fig.3.24**) Your fingers should never press directly onto the skin. Locate the blackhead you want to take out, then place your fingers around it and push up; rotate around the blackhead and push upward again. (**Fig. 3.25**) If the skin has been properly softened by the steam, the blackhead should come right out. Wipe the area gently with the tissue and refold it inward; dispose of the tissue after you have cleaned each small area. In general, it's best to clean only those blackheads that squeeze out easily; if a client complains that it hurts, you should stop. In some cases, if a blackhead is very hard to clean out, you can use a disposable sterilized needle to gently prick the pore and then squeeze it out very gently. Not all estheticians feel comfortable with this method, and it is essential to exercise caution. Whiteheads should never be squeezed; they can be poked gently, right on top, using a sterile disposable needle. (**Fig. 3.26**) In each case, a new needle should be used for each blemish and all needles should be

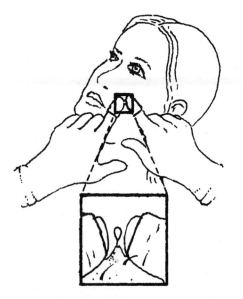

Fig. 3.25. Apply gentle pressure around the blackhead and push upward.

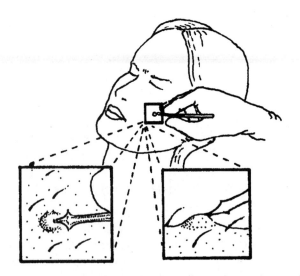

Fig. 3.26. A disposable, sterilized needle can be used to gently prick the pore.

disposed of immediately. In most cases, blackheads and whiteheads are clustered in the T-zone, on the nose and forehead. Occasionally, clogged pores may also develop along the hairline or behind the ears; hairsprays or mousses that clog the pores are often to blame.

Along with being extragentle in squeezing the pores, there are certain key rules you should observe during the pore-cleansing process:

- *Never* squeeze blackheads inside the ears. This should be done by a physician (preferably a dermatologist) only.

- *Never* clean whiteheads near the eyes. The risks are too great that you could damage the delicate tissue or accidentally poke someone in the eye.

- Be careful not to overdo the pore-cleansing process. Every skin will eventually become sensitive if it is pushed or picked at enough, so it is vital that an esthetician observe her client's skin's limits. If a client has not had a thorough skin cleaning recently and there are a great many blackheads, then it is the esthetician's responsibility to inform the client that it would be best to do some pore cleaning today and then return for an additional cleaning in a few weeks, to avoid irritating the skin. If you explain to clients that this way redness and extreme irritation can be avoided, they usually appreciate the honesty and will be happy to come back sooner. In any case, the importance of not overdoing pore cleansing is each esthetician's responsibility; don't let a pushy client press you into doing so much that the skin is left red and blotchy.

- Even under the best of circumstances, pore cleansing can be an uncomfortable process. Therefore, it's crucial that the esthetician keep monitoring client comfort, assuring the client that if at any point the cleansing process hurts, you will stop.

- *Never* attempt to clean out cystic, infected acne lesions. In the case of an isolated acne breakout, use **peroxide** to cleanse the area thoroughly and then apply **sulfa powder** to the skin, covered with a dab of a mud mask to hold it in place. This will at least have a calming effect on the blemish.

The Final Step of Pore Cleansing

After cleansing the pores, sterilize the skin by applying peroxide all over the face, using a square of sterilized cotton to apply it. Next, apply a liquid cleansing lotion or astringent, depending on the skin type.

THE MASK: A THREE-STEP SKIN IMPROVEMENT

The next step in most facials is the application of a facial mask; the most luxurious facials include more than one mask. The best facial includes three masks: therapeutic, surface peeling, and calming.

The Therapeutic Mask

The first mask is a **therapeutic** mask, so to speak, geared to the type of skin each client has. If the skin is dry, choose an herb-formula mask. If the skin is dry but needs some cleansing in the T-zone, a gel mask that will tighten a little bit more is a good choice. For oily skin, a mud mask is a good choice; for very oily skin, a clay mask is even better. On combination skin, you might apply a mud mask on the T-zone and a **herb-based** or **egg-and-honey** mask on the cheeks. If a client has mild acne, apply a **camphor-based** mask to the T-zone and a mud or clay mask on the cheeks.

Whatever formula you choose, apply the mask with a spatula (never with your hands) in a thin layer; cotton pads dipped in cool water should cover the eyes and the mask should never be applied near the eyes. (**Fig. 3.27**) If the neck area is dry, this is a good time to apply a neck cream.

A mask should be left on for seven to eight minutes—no longer. It's a good idea to stay in the room for the first one to two minutes to be sure that the client is comfortable and that the

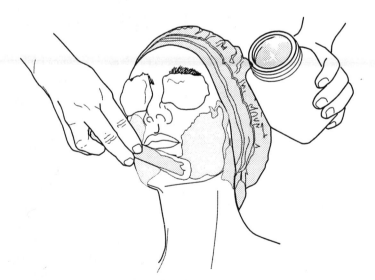

Fig. 3.27. Use a spatula to apply the mask.

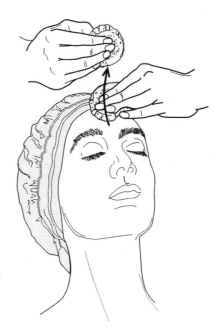

Fig. 3.28. Use one piece of cotton per stroke, then discard; otherwise, you will simply be brushing the mask back onto the skin.

mask doesn't sting or burn; if the client tells you it's uncomfortable, you should remove the mask right away.

Use warm water on cotton to remove the mask. Always use gentle upward-moving strokes, moving up from the jawline to the cheeks. Use each cotton pad for one complete stroke and then throw it away and use a new one; otherwise, you will simply be brushing the mask back onto the skin. (**Fig. 3.28**)

The Surface Peeling Mask

The second mask is a gentle **surface peeling** mask to cleanse away any dead cells. It should be applied in a very thin layer, kept well away from the eyes or the mouth, and removed within two minutes. Before cleaning the mask off, wash your hands and gently massage the mask into the skin. Then use cotton and warm water to remove the mask, again using an upward sweeping stroke of the cotton.

The Calming Mask

The third mask is in some ways the most important one, because it will help determine how the skin looks at the end of the facial. This mask should be a **calming** mask, to help soothe the skin and leave it looking fresh. A **calamine-powder/ yogurt** mask is one good choice, as is any **antiseptic-formula** mask. In some salons, a **seaweed** or **sea algae** mask is offered at an additional charge. If skin is a little irritated, using very cool compresses on the face as a mask in themselves is a good choice. Simply take cotton, dip it in cool water, and make three long pads. Place one across the cheeks, one across the forehead, and the last along the jawline. Take small ice cubes and go over the pads with them to keep the mask cool.

The most important rule of any professional facial is that the skin should never be left red and blotchy. This point cannot be overemphasized, because it is the number-one reason people use to avoid facials in the first place—and is the way that overzealous facialists can give the whole profession a bad name. If the skin is left red and blotchy, it means that the esthetician either squeezed too many blackheads, squeezed the skin too forcefully, or used the wrong products for that client's skin type. Too many clients are fearful of thorough skin cleansing because they were left scarred—often quite literally—by poorly trained facialists. For this reason, if there is any redness or blotchiness at this point, it is up to you to use the cold mask previously outlined to relieve it.

After removing the final mask, spray on a mist of skin-freshening spray (a mineral water spray, or papaya- or aloe-based freshener, perhaps). Then take a tissue and gently blot the skin so it doesn't feel wet. Ask clients if their eyes feel comfortable or if they'd like a cool cotton wash. Then apply moisturizer all over the face and, if the client approves it, eye cream.

SHOULDER MASSAGE: ENDING UP RELAXED

This is the point at which many standard facials end. But for a truly relaxing finishing touch, a gentle shoulder massage is a highly polished way to complete the salon experience. First, sit the client up by slowly raising the chair back. Sprinkle a small amount of talcum powder on the shoulders and neck so that any remaining lotions will be absorbed and won't stain the client's clothes once they're put back on. Take the heel of each hand and roll gently over each shoulder to help take the kinks out. Using three fingers—the pointer, middle finger, and ring finger— of each hand, gently lift each side of the neck, rubbing from the base of the neck upward to the jawline. Do this two or three times, then ask the client to look in the mirror and see how relaxed and refreshed the results are. (**Figs. 3.29, 3.30**)

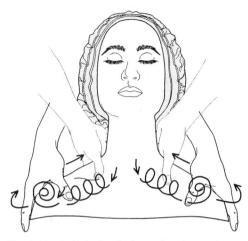

Fig. 3.29. Roll the heel of your hand over the shoulders.

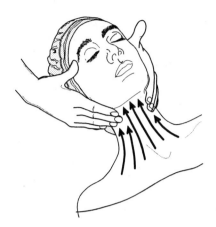

Fig. 3.30. Use the middle, ring, and pointer fingers to lift each side of the neck.

It is standard at this point to inform female clients that a makeup room or makeup artist is available. It is important, though, not to push makeup on a client, as some may simply want to leave the skin fresh and clean. The makeup should be offered, but the decision should be left up to the client. In most cases, simply applying eye makeup and some lipstick is really the best choice, because this allows the skin to breathe freely after the facial treatment.

SELF-QUIZ: QUESTIONS TO CONSIDER

In many salons, rock music is played throughout the treatment rooms and reception area. Is this appropriate?

Author's Advice: Music is a wonderfully stimulating and relaxing part of visiting a skin care salon, but it should be chosen carefully. As a general rule, music should not be too loud, because one of the primary benefits of a facial is its relaxing effect. Rock music is one possible choice, if it is appropriate to a particular salon's clientele, but it should be soft rock rather than heavy metal. (Even those who like hard rock would have to agree that it is not usually relaxing!) Classical music is one of the best choices, as it is generally easy to listen to for everyone (obviously, Chopin is a better choice than a Wagner opera). Many salons simply choose a local classical music station and play it softly throughout the salon; then there is no worry about remembering to change records or cassettes.

Facial masks sometimes seem hard to remove without some vigorous rubbing of the skin. Is this a frequent problem?

Author's Advice: One problem is that some estheticians leave masks on the skin for too long. As noted in this chapter's section dealing with masks, the longest time any mask should be left on the skin is five to eight minutes; even a minute or two longer and it can harden on the skin. A mask that's left to harden becomes hard to remove without vigorous rubbing at the skin, increasing the chances of irritation.

Another reason that masks may be hard to remove is that the cotton used to remove them isn't soft enough or isn't dipped in warm water. Be sure that the water is warm, not cold, and you will have to rub much less at the skin.

It's also important that you be especially gentle whenever you rub a product onto or off of the skin. Better to have to repeat the mask-cleansing process than to have rubbed too hard and left the skin reddened or irritated.

Many European-trained estheticians use sponges on the skin. Aren't these the most natural choice?

Author's Advice: Sponges are a wonderful choice if a salon can afford to throw them away after each client. Since this isn't practical, using sterilized cotton is a better choice, since it is extra-gentle on the skin and can be used only once and then thrown away. Although the chance that sponges will spread bacteria may be lessened greatly by washing them thoroughly with hot water and soap and leaving them out in the air to dry, it is better to be safe than sorry. For this reason, sterile cotton, cut into two-inch squares with scissors that have been sterilized, is a better choice.

CHAPTER 4   Special Facials

In this chapter, you will learn how to give eleven different facials that go beyond the basics. Each facial is intended for a specific skin type and for clients for whom spending a bit of extra money for additional attention, pampering, and skin care is an important part of the salon experience. Here's what you will find on the following pages:

- eleven different facials that are targeted to specific skin types—dry, oily, mature, and extrasensitive
- a special anti-stress skin treatment
- the reasons *not* to fall for minifacials
- spot treatments aimed at specific areas of the face.

Most salons offer at least one or two special facials. Often, a new salon will concentrate on supplying the basics, as well as one or two special treatments, then add other treatments as the salon clientele grows and new products and facial machines come onto the market. The prices charged to clients vary, but usually range from the same price as a regular facial (for treatments that may just involve adding or substituting for one step of a regular facial) to twice the standard price. Because these treatments do involve additional cost to the client, it is important not to push them on anyone, but simply to let clients know that they are available via brochure listings or unpressured discussions. Frequently it is the client who expresses a desire for something special, either as a result of wanting to know if anything more can be done to reduce, for example, skin oiliness or dryness, or of becoming interested in taking even better care of the skin.

The facials described in this chapter combine real skin benefits with the latest in skin care ingredients and facial machines. In most cases, they involve substituting a special treatment for the last mask of the basic facial, so you will not find every step of the facial outlined here, only the one or two additional steps.

51

FOR DRY SKIN

There are three types of masks that, substituted for the last mask of a basic facial (as described in chapter 3), give an added degree of moisturizing to skin that is dry or flaky.

Paraffin Wax Treatment

This mask is intended for skin that is very dry but that is not overly heat sensitive and does not have broken capillaries or excessive sun damage. It should be used as the last mask of a three-mask facial.

In a special paraffin "bath" machine, melt paraffin containing mixed vegetable and essential oils. (Never use a pot of paraffin; the machine makes sure that the melted oils never become dangerously hot.) Always be sure that the client's hair is protected with a headband or turban-towel wrap and that the eyes are covered with damp sterile cotton. To protect the skin and boost moisturization, apply **vitamin E cream** to the skin first, then brush on four coats of the paraffin, using a one-inch-wide, very soft paintbrush. Use a downward brush stroke, starting at the forehead and going down the face. (**Fig. 4.1**) If the client's lips are dry, the paraffin can even be applied to the lips over a coat of lip balm (ask first before applying, though, as some clients

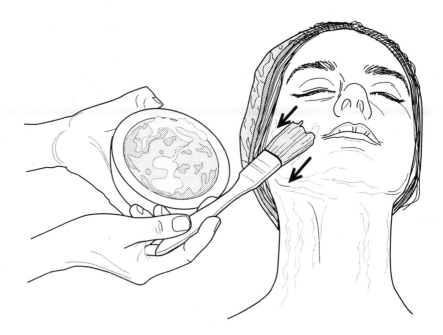

Fig. 4.1. Use a one-inch paintbrush with downward strokes.

become nervous if the whole face is covered). The beauty of paraffin is that it helps everything that is applied underneath to penetrate more deeply, because it holds in and reflects body heat. In essence, the paraffin becomes a mini-sauna for the face.

The mask can be left on for up to ten minutes, but before you leave the room, ask if the client is comfortable. Some clients may feel a bit closed in with a paraffin mask, so it's a good idea to return to the facial room every few minutes to check that everything is all right and to remove the mask if the client feels uncomfortable.

SPOTLIGHT
....

As a skin care specialist, you never know where you will find your inspiration for new services to offer. In the case of my own salon, I got my start in doing special facials through one of my most loyal clients, who had followed me from one salon to another when I was an employee and had then joined me as my very first patron once I opened my own salon. After about a year at my salon, she came in one day and said to me, "Lia, I love what your facials do for my skin, but I keep reading in magazines about different kinds of facials at other places. I think I'm getting a little bored with the same old thing. I don't want to leave you, but isn't there something else you could do for my skin?"

Well, I certainly didn't want to lose one of my most long-standing clients. I had to think fast. It occurred to me that the company that manufactured the paraffin bath machine we used for hand treatments had told me it also made a machine for use with facials, in a slightly smaller size. Because my client had dry skin, I knew that the same principle of moisturization would apply to her facial skin as it would to the skin of the hands. She was also using collagen ampoules as a once-a-week night "cream," and I knew she liked the results. After thinking for a minute, I said to her, "How about an extra-moisturizing collagen ampoule facial?" Her answer, "Wow. That sounds great."

Right then and there, I came up with the idea of applying the collagen ampoule under a thin layer of paraffin as the final mask in a facial. When I saw how much her skin benefited, and how much she loved the results, I decided to call the paraffin-machine company right after she left the salon to order the facial machine. Over the next few months, I experimented with the technique on myself and my salon staff and eventually came up with the precise application of four thin coats of paraffin to get the most moisturizing possible.

I also learned another important lesson that day: As with anything in life, getting the same old facial every month or two can become boring. As a salon owner, it's my job to come up with new ideas *before* any of my clients get bored!

The paraffin will lift cleanly off the face in a single piece when you are ready to remove it. Always throw it away immediately; *never* reuse paraffin.

The Intensive Treatment

This facial is intended for dry, mature skin. It combines a revved-up **collagen** mask with the use of **galvanic current** to help soften fine lines and reactivate the skin's natural elasticity so that it acts younger. It is also a good choice for those who have very dry skin due to skiing or swimming in chlorinated pools. Clients usually feel that it boosts the effects of a facial on their skin, keeping the skin looking fresher for several weeks, as opposed to a week or so after the treatment.

This treatment begins with a basic facial. A light peeling mask is used as the second mask. As the third mask, a mixture of soluble **collagen powder** is mixed with a **collagen ampoule** (this boosts the collagen percentage from 5 percent to 15 percent) and then applied wherever the skin is dry on the face and neck. Galvanic current is then applied using the **galvanic machine** (as described in chapter 5). The current from this machine boosts the skin's absorption of the collagen, deeply hydrating the skin and boosting its suppleness. (**Fig. 4.2**)

The Supergentle Moisturizer

There are some people whose skin is not only very dry but also easily irritated by virtually anything that's applied to it—heat, machines, product ingredients. In this case, you need to exercise great care both in cleansing the skin and in using masks. For these clients, the last mask of a three-mask facial should be warm **cod liver** or **olive oil**, both of which are especially gentle and will help to soothe skin after gentle cleansing. Soak pieces of cotton in the warm (not hot) oil and then squeeze out the pieces and apply them over the face (avoiding the eye area, of course, which should be covered with cool compresses). To boost the skin penetration of the oil, you can use an **infrared lamp** set on low and positioned about a foot away from the face (the client's eyes *must* be covered with damp compresses). Leave the oil on the skin for ten minutes, then use warm, damp cotton to cleanse off excess oil. (**Fig. 4.3**)

Retin-A: Dry, Sensitive Skin

As **Retin-A** has become more popular as a medical treatment for both acne and aging skin, the number of clients who show up at skin care salons with the dry, slightly irritated results has also increased. For this reason, top salons have to develop facial methods that will not add to the side effects from the use

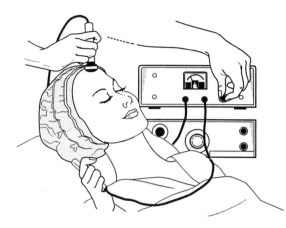

Fig. 4.2. The galvanic machine. The client must hold one probe while the other is used on the skin.

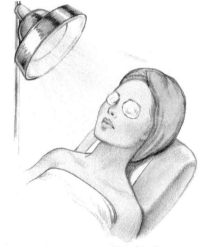

Fig. 4.3. Leave oil on the skin for ten minutes while using the infrared lamp; remove with warm, damp cotton.

of this drug, which makes the skin surface very sensitive. As an esthetician, you must be on the lookout for clients who use Retin-A, as you do not want to unknowingly irritate their complexions. A good skin history should always include the question of whether the client uses any medications, in pill or topical form, for the skin.

When giving a facial to someone who uses Retin-A, steaming should be kept to a minimum (roughly half the usual time is a good idea) and the amount of gentle massage and cream should be increased. Before steaming, you can apply a mixture of vitamin E, olive oil, and cod liver oil; it will usually soak right into the skin and help protect it from the steam. As the last mask, you can use a **calamine powder** mask, which is very calming, or a **seaweed algae** mask (usually provided at an extra charge). It is also important to encourage clients who use Retin-A to apply moisturizer daily.

FOR OILY SKIN

Here are three different ideas for facials that help control skin oiliness and also discourage breakouts.

Yeast Mask

If skin is excessively oily, it is a good idea to skip the massage that is usually given during a basic facial and to concentrate on cleaning out impurities; then follow up with a **yeast mask/**

lemon-sugar cleanser. After cleaning the pores, apply a mixture of lemon juice (for an antiseptic effect) and sugar (a natural cleanser) all over the face, then cover the face with a tissue and apply a yeast mask over the tissue. (This layered effect allows the lemon and sugar to do their jobs before the yeast mask seeps through, making this a "time-release" treatment.) After ten minutes, remove the tissue, taking the yeast with it, and cleanse the face.

Seaweed Treatment

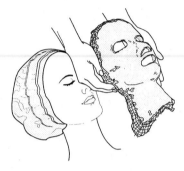

Fig. 4.4. The seaweed mask will lift off the skin in one piece.

For oily skin that seems clogged and has a great many blackheads, the detoxifying effect of a final seaweed mask is recommended. Seaweed retains solar energy, natural vitamins, minerals, and amino acids, and so helps restore needed balance to many skin types, especially oily skin. As the final mask, mix seaweed powder with milk (also rich in amino acids and a good skin calmer) to make a paste and apply to skin. Leave on for ten minutes and then remove by simply lifting the mask off the skin (it should lift off very easily if the paste has been mixed and applied properly). (**Fig. 4.4**) This mask can also be used for combination skin: just apply it in the T-zone and then apply a collagen mask, for example, to the rest of the face.

Electronic Skin Improvement Machines

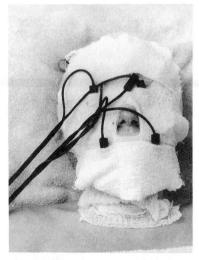

Fig. 4.5. The electronic probe machine. (Courtesy of Steve Victor, M.D.)

For oily skin, the electronic probe machine helps unclog pores, reduce enlarged pores, and rebalance the skin's oil output through the use of special cosmetic solutions applied to the face along with low-grade electrical currents. This skin care system is a four-month treatment regimen, with between one and four salon treatments a week; the treatment itself takes approximately twenty minutes.

The treatment is not exceedingly complicated. The skin is cleansed thoroughly using a special cleanser that helps maintain the skin's natural surface chemistry. Then an electrolyzed cosmetic solution (as determined by skin type) is sprayed onto the skin, which is then covered with a terry cloth/gauze mask that has pockets into which special probes are placed. (**Fig. 4.5**) The machine is then programmed to emit a specific current level, depending on the degree of skin damage. Some people report skin improvement after just one treatment; others require four or five before significant improvement is noticeable.

CAUTION: Because this treatment involves the use of low-level electricity, it shouldn't be used on pregnant women, or anyone with a pacemaker or who has epilepsy.

ABOUT COSTS: Because these treatments are usually expensive, and require some education of the client before a commitment is made, it is customary at the best salons to offer a free consultation about the treatment specifics.

ANTI-STRESS TREATMENTS

The Relaxation Facial

For many clients, stress is what they come to the skin care salon to "treat." It's what makes their skin look less than fresh and makes them feel older than their years. For these clients, one can develop an antistress facial that, more than any other, puts the emphasis on relaxation. The difference: instead of spending ten minutes massaging the face, as you would in a basic facial, take twenty-five minutes to repeat the whole massage procedure at least twice through. Right after the first cleansing, before you apply the steam machine, smooth a mixture of **azulene** and **papaya** soothing masks onto the face and gently massage it into the skin while the steam is running. During the facial, constantly take short breaks to massage the neck and shoulders, either while a mask is setting or in between steps of the facial. Put the emphasis on relaxation in everything you, as the esthetician, do, and your clients will appreciate it as you give them a chance to take a little vacation from stress right in the salon.

Hand Massage

This is a de-stressing treatment that can easily be added to any type of facial. In some salons, mini–hand treatments are offered as a part of every facial; in others, they are given as a special every-other-facial treat or offered at a small additional charge. Here is a seven-step hand massage that targets areas of the hand where people really tend to "hold onto" stress:

1. **Hand Shake.** Hold the client's hands level with the chest and shake them vigorously to a count of twenty-five. This warms up and limbers the hands at the same time that it increases circulation.

2. **Cream Massage.** Starting with the palms, massage a rich hand cream into the client's hands, being sure to rub it in as much as possible, so that the skin is smoothed. Then apply more hand cream to your own hands so that, as you give the following steps of the massage, you are automatically applying more hand cream to the client.

3. **Open/Close Movement.** Starting with the right hand, take the client's hand in your own and close it as a fist. Hold it tight, gently squeezing it (don't press too hard, especially if the client has long nails!) to a count of five, then release. Repeat with left hand, then alternate hands five more times. This exercise helps to strengthen and stretch the hand muscles.

4. **Palm Work.** Bring the client's hands together, palms facing each other, in front of the chest, as if in prayer. Then bend the clasped hands to the left, then to the right. In a gentle rhythm, bend back and forth to a count of twenty. This exercise strengthens the hands and wrists and makes them more flexible.

5. **Finger Play.** Starting with the thumb of the client's right hand, massage each finger separately by rubbing each finger from the knuckle slowly up to the tip. Repeat on left hand; then go back to right hand and do again, finishing up a second time on the left hand. (As you massage, dip your own fingers back into the hand cream, so that you are keeping the moves smooth and soft.) This exercise helps stimulate circulation and relax the hands.

6. **Wrist Circles.** Hold one hand on the client's right wrist and the other on the right hand. Gently circle the hand in the air to a count of twenty. Reverse and repeat. Then repeat in two directions with the left hand. This exercise helps to keep the wrists limber.

7. **Smooth Finish.** To complete the treatment, apply more hand cream, then cover the client's hands in plastic bags and put them into heated **mitts** for two to three minutes to enhance the skin absorption of the moisturizing ingredients. (See Fig. 5.5, page 71)

MINIFACIALS: WHY THEY'RE A HOAX

In this time-pressed world, everything that can be done faster is offered as an advance. Skin care is no exception and today many salons offer so-called minifacials, promising to have their clients in and out in thirty minutes flat. Though the promise sounds great, they don't deliver results. Offering these facials is unprofessional and a disservice to clients.

For one thing, it takes about twenty minutes for the skin to achieve the softness and pliability needed to really be cleaned efficiently. You cannot steam a client's skin for one minute, cleanse it for five minutes, offer three minutes of massage and a five-minute mask and expect to have done the skin much good at all. In fact, most half-hour facials leave the skin red and blotchy-looking because the esthetician is trying to do as much as possible to the skin in as little time as possible.

When you consider how much time it takes you to do your job correctly—roughly five to seven minutes to do the initial cleansing of the skin surface before even beginning to clean the pores, a full minute or more to gently apply a mask, a good five to ten minutes of massage before the client even begins to relax—you will see how difficult it is to deliver anything approaching good skin care in half an hour. Nevertheless, the money that can be made by packing as many facials as possible into a single day continues to drive many entrepreneurs to offer minifacials.

A good, thorough facial takes one hour and fifteen minutes. If a client is in a rush, by trimming some time from the massage and mask time, it's possible to whittle this down to forty-five to fifty minutes. But in less than that time, the benefits to the clients are significantly reduced, while the price they pay—in money and roughly handled skin—is too high. In most cases, a facial that is done too quickly shows up on the client's face, in the form of skin irritation or blotchiness, because the skin does not have time to recover between the steps of the facial. Clients who leave the salon quickly but not looking their best aren't the type of client you want.

SPOT TREATMENTS

For many people, aging isn't an all-at-once process. It usually starts in one or more key areas of the face: around the eyes, around the lips, or on the neck. For these people, you can offer smaller (and less expensive) versions of the Ionic Facial Toning Lift (discussed in chapter 9) by targeting the treatment only to one area.

Eye Energizer

Utilize the Ionic Facial Toning Lift machine around the eyes only for a ten-minute treatment that will seem to take years off a client's face. Before using the machine, be sure to cleanse the area using an extragentle gel cleanser and apply an eye cream suited to the client's skin type and degree of skin damage.

Mouth Smoother

It is especially common for smokers to age quickly around their mouths, since the constant pursing of their lips around cigarettes etches in lines and wrinkles. By using the Ionic Facial Toning Lift machine only around the mouth for a ten-minute treatment, you can add an additional low-cost feature to a basic facial. Apply a lightweight moisturizer around the mouth first, or use a collagen ampoule for a more intensive treatment.

Neck Lift

Sun damage can make a person's neck look more wrinkled than the face or the rest of the body. To target this area, you can use the Ionic Facial Toning Lift machine for ten minutes intensively on the neck, concentrating on those areas where skin has become lax, wrinkled, or crepey-looking.

SELF-QUIZ: QUESTIONS TO CONSIDER

I have heard that the Ionic Facial Toning Lift is also offered by dermatologists. Are these medical treatments better?

Author's Advice: In actuality, they are the same treatments, using the same machine to stimulate the skin with cotton-tipped probes and a mild, pulsating current. The fact is, though, that dermatologists—as well as plastic surgeons and chiropractors, many of whom also offer this treatment—usually charge more for this type of nonsurgical facelift than do skin care salons.

Of course, there is no need to build animosity between skin care experts and medical personnel; it is really up to the individual client where to go for various skin services. In fact, many of my own clients consult with dermatologists as well as coming to my salon for treatments—and I even work with their dermatologists or plastic surgeons to help deliver the best possible results. It is best to simply explain to clients that the same type of treatment is offered at various places, to explain your own expertise and the type of follow-up advice you can offer, and then to allow the client to decide.

Since it's customary in many salons to work on more than one client at a time, I'm worried that I might have to leave a mask on for more than ten minutes. Is there any danger to the client's skin?

Author's Advice: Most masks can easily be left on the skin for between ten and fifteen minutes without doing the skin any harm. In fact, in the case of a deep-moisturizing or soothing mask, you might want to leave it on for twelve minutes or so rather than ten to give it a little more time to do its job. What you do want to avoid, though, is ever leaving any type of mask on for longer than fifteen minutes. Depending on the ingredients, it could become either irritating or harden onto the skin, making it more difficult to remove. A mask that is difficult to remove requires rubbing at the skin during the cleansing-off step, which increases the chance of skin irritation.

I have noticed that some salons push their clients, after a few visits, to consider "stepping up" to a special, more expensive type of facial. Is this proper?

Author's Advice: A hard sell is never the best idea in any type of business, but especially in one as personal as skin care. In fact, there is no need for anyone to have more than a basic facial at any time. Properly done, a basic facial can fulfill all of a client's skin care needs. For this reason, I believe that an esthetician may educate clients about the different types of facials available, but should never push them. This is best done by offering information, both in discussion and by giving the client a copy of a brochure if one is available in the salon. It is also customary in the best salons to offer free consultations about all services for first-time clients and to offer further consultations, also free of charge, for any client who is considering a new or different type of service, especially if it involves considerable expense. To do otherwise gives an overly pushy impression that reflects poorly not only on the individual skin care salon but on the profession as a whole.

CHAPTER 5

Salon Facial Equipment

In this chapter, you will become familiar with the basic equipment found in most skin care salons. Along with general descriptions of the types of equipment, you will also find:

- machines that are essential versus those that are a luxury
- tips on getting machines to work more efficiently or last longer
- advice on keeping machinery clean
- several machines that are more hype than help to a professional esthetician.

No brand names are listed in this chapter because it is not the intention of this book to help sell any specific manufacturer's machines. Magazines geared to estheticians regularly have advertisements featuring specific manufacturers' machines, and there is no shortage of "beauty shows" around the country at which different companies present their wares and extol the virtues of their equipment as compared to their competitors'. As an overall guide, keep in mind that, as with any machinery in recent years, computerized and high-tech advances are showing up in many types of facialist equipment. However, the more high tech the machine, the more complicated it often is to set up and use. A machine that requires too much of an esthetician's attention takes her attention away from her craft and her client, so the more advanced machine may not always be the best choice. If you're shopping for machines, shop carefully and take time to decide.

CHAIRS: MORE THAN JUST SOMETHING TO SIT ON

Whatever the colors or decor in most skin care salons, when it comes to the chairs used in the treatment rooms, the overwhelming choice is white, because it inspires a look of cleanliness and hygiene that is essential to the practice of high-quality skin care. Of course, like all other equipment in the salon, chairs must be scrubbed down regularly and kept scrupulously clean.

Reclining Chairs

Reclining chairs for the client come in two basic types: with arm-rests and without. Many salons offer both types. There are also varying degrees of softness in the upholstery; some are very soft and cushiony, others less so (the flatter, more "orthopedic"-type chairs, interestingly, are often preferred by male clients). The best advice is to purchase the best-made chair possible with several easily adjustable positions. Remember that the chair's degree of recline will have to be changed, depending on the treatments being given, several times during each facial, from sitting straight up to lying almost flat.

The chair must be fastidiously clean at all times. It should always be covered first by a sheet and then by a fresh towel that is changed for each individual client.

Stools

Although ideally stools should have backrests to protect your back, in most salons these aren't the type that are used. Most salon owners purchase backless stools because they're less expensive and also take up less room. What is essential, though, is that the stools have wheels, so that the esthetician can move easily around the room and not make noise while shifting position during a facial. The stools should also be easily adjustable in height, as no two operators or clients will be the same height. Many stools are shoddily made—a good one should last five to ten years.

GETTING A GOOD LOOK AT CLIENTS

The Magnifying Lamp

The magnifying lamp is one of the most essential tools for professional skin care, because it allows you to get a good, thorough look at each client's skin. A good lamp with strong, glare-free magnification and a high-quality light ensures that you can do a thorough assessment of the client's skin, and also gives a professional look to the salon. These same types of lamps are also regularly used by doctors, dermatologists, plastic surgeons, and operating rooms.

The bulb used in the lamp should always be plain white—a colored lamp gives the look of a disco, not a professional image. Clients' eyes should always be covered when you are examining their skin through the lamp, to avoid glaring the light into their eyes.

The type of magnifying lamp used in most salons is mounted on a stand on the floor. However, in many other salons the lamps are mounted on the wall. You must be very careful in

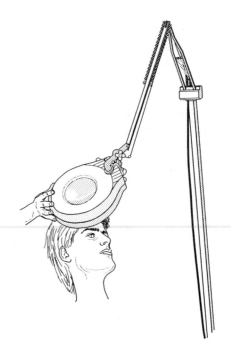

Fig. 5.1. The magnifying lamp.

using them, not only to avoid swinging the lamp into your or a client's head, but also to check the lamp's stability at the start of each day. Given the number of times each day that the lamp will be swung back and forth and up and down, it's not surprising that, over time, the bolts holding the lamp to the wall could loosen. Eventually, the result could be a very heavy lamp falling onto you or a client. Whatever the type of lamp, it should be cleaned and checked, just like the rest of your equipment, at the start of each work day to ensure that nothing feels loose. If it does, it's best to have the salon manager or someone else check the attachments and avoid using that facial room that day. Better to be safe than sorry. (**Fig. 5.1**)

TWIN ESSENTIALS: STEAMER AND HIGH-FREQUENCY MACHINE

The past few years have seen a wide introduction of machinery for use in giving facials. Some of the more specialized machines are featured in the chapter on special facials, but there are some that every esthetician should know how to use correctly. Two that no salon can really be without are the **steam machine** and the **high-frequency machine**.

Steam Machines

Steam machines provide a steady, lukewarm mist of water onto the skin in a temperature-controlled, safe manner. Some salons, in an effort to economize, use bowls of warm to hot water and towels draped over the clients' heads as a substitute, but this method cannot provide the same controlled steaming of a machine, nor can it provide the same relaxation, because a client must sit up over the bowl (although it's fine for home treatments). In addition, it is far too easy to make the water too hot, with the result that the steam is so hot that it makes the client uncomfortable or, worse yet, feel almost scalded. Standard vaporizers meant for home use also are not a good substitute, because the steam that comes out can also be too hot and does not come out in as fine a vapor mist as a good facial steaming machine.

A professional steam machine, correctly positioned about fifteen inches from the skin surface, provides a lukewarm mist diffused over the skin. Benefits include:

- softening dead surface cells
- opening and softening follicles so that they can easily be cleaned of oil, makeup, and dirt
- softening blackheads so that they are easier to remove
- helping pores to eliminate toxins
- increasing circulation by causing local blood vessels to expand. (CAUTION: This can be a danger to anyone with already broken capillaries.) (**Fig. 5.2**)

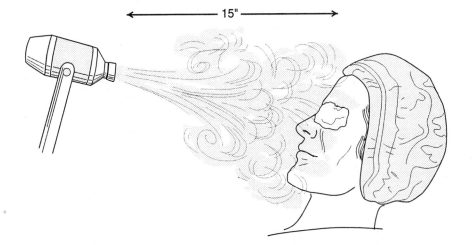

Fig. 5.2. The steam machine should be placed fifteen inches from the face.

Steam machines come in different models. Older versions need to warm up before being used; newer models turn off automatically, either with a timer or when the water level becomes low. If a machine has a glass reservoir but does not turn off automatically, it is imperative to check the water level several times during the day to avoid running the machine while empty; this can eventually crack the glass and burn up the machine.

To care for a steam machine properly, use *only* distilled or purified water. Tap water will provide satisfactory steam at first, but over time the machine will malfunction because of a buildup of calcium and other minerals. If you accidentally use tap water in the steam machine, clean it out with a plain vinegar and water solution, letting it run for several hours so that the minerals are thoroughly cleansed away.

Like any piece of equipment, even the best steam machine can break down or run hotter or cooler than normal. Cool mist is no danger, but too-hot mist can irritate or even burn a client's skin. Before leaving the room, always wait a few minutes to be sure that the client is comfortable, that the steam is not too hot, and that the vapor is covering the client's whole face. Be sure to cover the client's eyes with a cool compress before turning the machine toward the face, and keep the distance, as stated earlier, about fifteen inches between face and machine. One exception may be during summer, when the air conditioning is on strongly, which can cause the steam to cool down before it reaches the client at this distance. In that case, you may need to move the machine slightly closer.

High-Frequency Machines

An essential tool, the high-frequency machine truly disinfects the skin after a facial that has involved a good deal of pore cleansing. It can also be used for back facials and scalp treatments. If there is one high-tech machine to have in every salon, this is it.

Made of glass, these machines come in **mushroom or horseshoe shapes** and give off a violet or orange-red colored light (both colors produce the same effect). Although these machines are often given the nickname of "ultra rays" or "violet rays," they are not to be confused with ultraviolet light, which is hazardous to skin. They give off **infrared light** in varying degrees of intensity that can be adjusted via buttons on the machine. These infrared rays have the benefit of completely disinfecting the skin and avoiding the accidental spread of infection, as well as stimulating circulation and glandular activity, increasing metabolism, and aiding deeper penetration of products into the skin. (**Figs. 5.3, 5.4**)

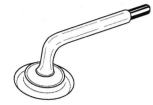

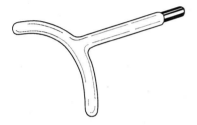

Fig. 5.3. Mushroom- and horseshoe-shaped high-frequency machines.

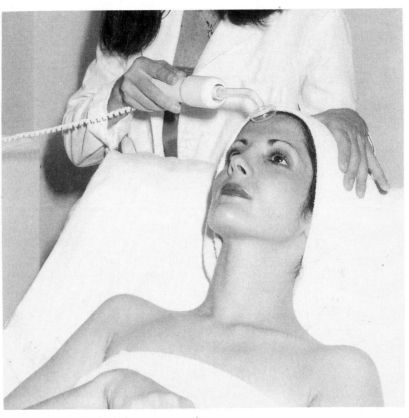

Fig. 5.4. Using the high-frequency machine.

For safety, no machine should ever be used on wet skin or on any woman who is pregnant. The machine itself must be sterilized with alcohol before each client to avoid the risk of spreading infection. If you are in doubt as to whether the machine has been sterilized, do it again.

If only one machine can be purchased for a salon, this is the one to get because it is the most efficient skin disinfectant and heightens the benefits of pore-cleansing facials.

EUROPE VERSUS AMERICA: MACHINE CHIC

In Europe, even the smallest skin care salon often has a multitude of machines, used for everything from cleansing to energizing to "deionizing" the skin. From the time a European woman gets her first facial, she is exposed to this machinery, and thus expects it as part of a good facial. By contrast, American skin care has taken a very hands-on approach—it is the power of the esthetician, not just the machinery, that gets the results.

In many American salons, machinery is kept to an absolute minimum—just a steam machine for facials and no other equipment save a wax-melter for use in hair removal. In others, the European machine ethic has been fully adopted, and it sometimes seems as if the esthetician's hands rarely touch the clients' faces. The use of too many machines, though, can remove the personal touch, and the pampering, from skin caring, which seems a bit counterproductive. In some cases, machinery is used to give a sophisticated aura to a salon that doesn't offer very high-quality services. Though that may work in attracting clients at first, eventually it will backfire. What keeps clients coming back consistently to a salon are the personnel and the pampering and quality of service. All the machinery in the world won't substitute for that.

In salons where a mixture of personal touch and high-quality machinery is the aim, three machines are often part of the essential facial equipment:

1.   the heat lamp
2.   the galvanic machine
3.   hot mitts

The Heat Lamp

Commonly called **infrared**, this lamp is used to produce heat that increases product penetration without increasing body temperature. It is valuable in keeping skin healthy, especially when special creams are applied or oil treatments are being given to extremely dry skin. In salons in which scalp treatments are offered, the infrared lamp can also be used to encourage penetration of scalp-moisturizing masks or creams.

CAUTION: Infrared lamps *do* get hot, so they must be positioned sufficiently far away from the client's face or scalp to avoid any danger of overheating or burning the skin. A distance of about twenty-five inches (a little more than two feet) is usually advised.

The Galvanic Machine

A galvanic machine has two important functions during facial treatments:

1.   to introduce water-soluble ingredients into the skin;
2.   to produce, through a very low-voltage constant, direct current, positive chemical reactions within the skin itself.

The machine itself consists of two **probes**—one positively charged, one negatively charged—that are attached to an electrical generator of sorts. There are several different types of machines, most of them imported from Europe during the past decade (galvanic treatments first became popular in Europe roughly twenty years ago). Some are, of course, more expensive than others, but they are all pretty much the same. The positive probe soothes nerves, decreases blood supply, and helps harden tissues; its power is used to help close pores, decrease skin redness, or help solutions penetrate into the skin. The negative probe stimulates nerves, increases blood supply, and softens tissues; its power is used to help stimulate blood circulation to the skin. That, of course, is the theory behind the electrical charges. In reality, the machine's biggest role is to help solutions penetrate more deeply into the skin.

When the machine is used, the negative probe is held in the client's hand and the positive probe, covered with cotton and the special solution, is placed on the client's skin, usually starting at the chin. The machine is then turned on, with the voltage on a low setting, and the probe is usually turned clockwise on the skin, covering a small area at a time and keeping the probe turning in a circle. Each time the probe is to be moved, it must be removed from the skin. The machine must be turned off and then turned on again once the probe is back on the skin. (See Fig. 4.2, page 55)

The total treatment usually takes at least ten minutes but will vary depending on a client's skin condition. The esthetician who uses this machine should be well trained and experienced in its use—and by this is meant not only in giving the treatment to others but in receiving it herself. If an esthetician has not experienced this treatment, she cannot really describe how it feels to someone else and can't be reassuring about its safety or its benefits. Some clients are very skeptical of machines and, although they want the benefits of a given treatment, worry about whether machines can hurt their skin. An esthetician who has used a machine can describe in a more personal manner what it feels like.

CAUTION: Galvanic machines should never be used on pregnant women, nor should they be used over broken capillaries or on very sensitive skin.

The galvanic machine should only be used by those who have been properly trained in its use, and should always be used on the lowest setting first, to be increased in tiny intervals

SPOTLIGHT

When I was an employee at a skin care salon that offered various types of machine treatments, it was often difficult for me to explain how the machines felt to my clients. I couldn't find the right words to describe the sensations they might feel, and my efforts to reassure them about a machine's value or safety often felt unconvincing to me. The problem was that I myself had not experienced all of the various treatments available at the salon. Yet the salon manager had never asked me whether I had had the facials I was constantly giving to my clientele.

Out of this experience came my determination that, if I had my own salon, I would offer all of the employees sample treatments of every type of service offered. The reason would not be mere generosity but to provide the best possible service to my clientele. An esthetician who understands the thinking behind a skin care treatment and has also experienced it is much more able to describe it to her clients than is someone who must only imagine what a machine feels like.

if both the esthetician and the client are comfortable with it. Care must be taken not to use the machine on clients who have braces, as the current sometimes causes a tingling effect. Those who have caps may also feel the current slightly in their teeth, so it's wise to ask. For some clients, the use of any sort of electric machine makes them nervous, so treatments can also be given without the galvanic current (or consider giving them the collagen paraffin facial described in chapter 4).

As with any machine that comes in direct contact with the skin, it is crucial to keep the galvanic machine, including the probes and all attachments, clean and sterilized between uses and to disinfect the machine again before each use.

Hot Mitts

Electrically warmed mitts are an optional accessory that add a touch of luxury to a salon. Used to give a heated moisturizing treatment to clients' hands, they are relatively inexpensive but often a client favorite—especially in wintertime, when hands become dry.

Mitts basically work like small heating pads; they are plugged into an electrical outlet and set on low, medium, or high. The low setting is usually sufficient for just about every use, but the higher settings can become uncomfortably warm for many people. The client's hands are first creamed and massaged, then put into

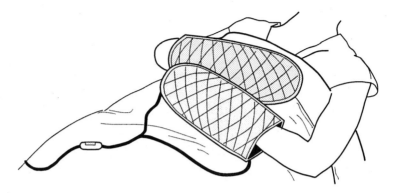

Fig. 5.5. Hot mitts.

tissues and then into clean plastic sandwich bags before being placed into the mitts. Some people can handle just five minutes of the heat treatment before they start feeling uncomfortably hot; others can go for twenty minutes. When the treatment is completed, you can let the hands cool inside the mitts, then remove the mitts and take off the tissues and plastic bags, which should then be thrown away. (Believe it or not, some salons actually try to reuse the plastic bags—an incredibly unsanitary practice.) (**Fig. 5.5**)

> CAUTION: As with any electrical appliance, the wiring of mitts should be checked regularly. Many mitts are cheaply made and can blow a fuse in the salon, plunging everyone into darkness. Most mitts can last for a year if used several times a day.

THE ESSENTIAL MACHINE: THE STERILIZER

A key machine in any salon is one that the vast majority of clients never see: the **sterilizer**, which is absolutely crucial in a world in which hygiene of beauty services is an increasing concern. Every salon should have a sterilizer to clean anything metal that is used—all manicure tools, tweezers, clippers, etc. The rated wattage of most sterilizing machines is 3.5 watts; the lamp voltage is 2 volts.

The sterilizing machine's key component is a **germicidal bulb** which, through heat and ultraviolet wavelengths, kills any microbes that could grow on salon implements. Because these tools come into direct contact with each client's skin,

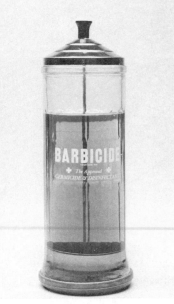

Fig. 5.6. Be sure to sanitize all tools.

whether on the face, hands, or body, they must be sterilized before every single use to avoid spreading infection from one client to another. All tools should be sterilized every morning and then resterilized between each treatment.

Even the best sterilizing machine is only as good as the care that every salon employee takes to use it. The implements should be washed thoroughly with soap and water first, then rinsed clean and dried with a freshly laundered towel (*never* reuse the drying towel, as it can also be a bacteria source). The implement should then be cleansed with alcohol and placed atop a clean tissue at the bottom of the sterilizing machine. The tools should be left in the sterilizer at least fifteen minutes to be sure that all germs have been killed. (**Fig. 5.6**)

The most important assessment that can be made of a salon's quality may be its rules of disinfecting. These practices indicate the seriousness with which the owner or manager views the health and safety of the employees as well as of the clients.

FACIAL GIMMICKRY: THREE MACHINES TO AVOID

As in any other field, the skin care profession is not immune to gimmicks. Quite often, these involve seemingly high-tech machines that do not provide any true benefit to the skin. In some cases, they can even be harmful. Three machines that have become quite popular are nevertheless quite questionable in their use.

Brushing Machines

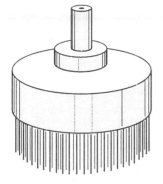

Fig. 5.7. Although it is claimed that these machines have a gentle vibrating action, they can be quite harsh on the skin, exerting much more pressure than a human hand using cloth.

Made in several sizes and shapes, some brushing machines are held by hand whereas others have a stand that holds the machinery on the floor. The stated purposes of brushing machines are to slough off dead cells and help in cleaning of the skin surface. They are usually used on the chin, forehead, and nose only, where it is claimed that skin is tough enough to take the action of the electric circling brush. (**Fig. 5.7**)

Although it is claimed that these machines have a gentle vibrating action, they can be quite harsh on the skin, exerting much more pressure than a human hand using a washcloth or sponge. Any brush's bristles can be harsh if pressed too hard onto delicate skin, and can be anathema to treating acne or skin that is aging or has a tendency to broken capillaries. The skin does not need to be rubbed or scrubbed at to become clean— it is a delicate, living material that can be injured. The pressure, roughness, and potential abrasiveness of facial brushes can

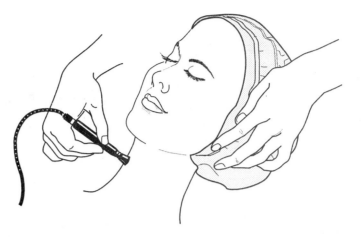

Fig. 5.8. The effect of the pulling action is really an illusion—and in fact cleans less thoroughly than careful, hands-on pore cleansing.

damage the elasticity of the skin, injure supportive fibers, and definitely spread infection if a client has any pimples on the skin surface or underneath.

In addition, facial brushes themselves can be a potential source of skin infection if they are not kept scrupulously clean. The brushes must be sterilized before and after every use—yet in many salons they are simply washed with soap and water.

Skin Vacuums

Suction machines also come with promises that can't necessarily be kept. These machines usually have various sizes of suction cups that are designed for use on different areas of the face during the cleansing process. By using these machines, it is claimed, an esthetician can pull dirt and oil out of the pores, offering a so-called deep-cleansing effect. (**Fig. 5.8**)

Although some people love the feeling of having their skin pulled at by these machines, the effect is really an illusion. The skin is cleaned no more deeply by being tugged at, and is in fact cleaned less thoroughly than by careful, hands-on pore cleansing. A vacuum is something to be used on a rug, not a person's face.

Spray Machines

These machines are not dangerous, but are certainly a bit of gimmickry that can add unnecessary expense to a salon's overhead—expense that often translates into higher prices for clients who are getting no advantage from this type of machinery.

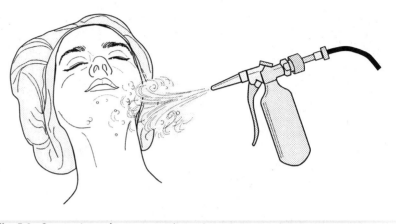

Fig. 5.9. Spray mister: the same result can be achieved with a simple pump bottle, at much less cost.

These machines are simply an electrified version of the pump-type mister that can be used to spray cooling mist onto the client's skin at the end of a facial. **(Fig. 5.9)**

There is no question that a cool misting of distilled water and a skin freshener at the end of a facial is a wonderful way to complete a skin treatment. But it is simple enough to use a pump bottle in which you have mixed two parts distilled water and one part skin freshener. If you want the effect of the superfine spray that some of these machines provide, simply place a tissue over the client's face as a spray filter, and then spray the freshener through the tissue. The effect produced will be exactly the same as using a machine that costs several hundred dollars.

SELF-QUIZ: QUESTIONS TO CONSIDER

I have heard claims that skin vacuums provide deep-cleansing benefits. Isn't this the case?

Author's Advice: Not at all. They provide the illusion, by pulling and tugging at the skin, that something significant is being done, when in fact the skin is simply being pulled and tugged at. The only way to truly provide deep cleansing is to take the time and effort to carefully clean the pores, using the hands-on approach described in chapter 3.

Many salons that I have visited do not seem to have sterilizing equipment. How necessary is this?

Author's Advice: In this day of increasing concerns about hygiene, a sterilizing machine is absolutely essential. If more estheticians refused to work in salons that did not sterilize their equipment, more salons would be forced to install this equipment. It is not even terribly costly, as most establishments would require only one machine.

CHAPTER 6

Body Basics: Skin Care from the Neck Down

With so much attention lavished on facial skin, both in the media and in salon treatments, it's easy to forget that professional skin care doesn't stop at the neck. In fact, some of the most luxurious skin treatments are now targeted to the body, and Americans are beginning to understand what Europeans have taken for granted for years: that well-cared-for skin should be a total-body concern, including the relaxation of massage and the specialized care of back "facials." Of course, taking care of body skin involves different concerns and requires different techniques than simply offering facials. In this chapter, you will learn:

- how to set up space for and offer back cleansing/moisturizing treatments
- the fine points of whether to offer massage in a salon, including staff and space requirements
- the ins and outs of body wraps, from seaweed to mud
- what you need to do about the two popular treatments of aromatherapy and reflexology, and whether to offer them to your clients.

BACK FACTS

The skin of the body, like that of the face, is constantly renewing itself. As new skin cells are produced, they move up to the surface to form the top layer of skin, then harden and die off to make way for new cells. Proper cleansing helps make this process more efficient, but few people pay attention to their body skin until dryness and flakiness—or blackheads and breakouts—appear. Even then, body skin care is not much of a tradition in America.

In the best salons, estheticians are always alert to helping their clients recognize the condition of the skin, not just on the face but on the body. During a facial, when a client is dressed in a robe, an esthetician should check the skin of the neck and of the back, and let the client know whether it is dry or oily and how best to care for body skin at home. If the skin is in need of a thorough cleansing or moisturizing, the esthetician should tell clients and inform them that such services are offered, at an additional charge, by the salon. A pushy sales job is not the intention; the client should be educated about the possibilities for body treatments but by no means pressured into having one right then and there. It's a good idea, in fact, to tell clients that such services are featured at the salon and offer them a pamphlet listing the full array of services when they are finished with their facials. That way, it is clear that it is up to the client to decide.

In fact, the back tends to be the oiliest part of the body, making it a major target for skin eruptions. Perspiration can be an additional culprit. The middle of the back (not the underarms) is often the first part of the body to start sweating during vigorous activity and exercise. The pores open, accumulated oil clogs the pores, and the result can be unsightly and uncomfortable blemishes. Many people who are well into their thirties and have relatively clear facial complexions find that they still suffer from blemishes on their backs.

A back "facial" is a relaxing and beneficial proposition. Properly done, it is as thorough a cleansing process as a traditional facial done on the face. First and foremost, though, a salon must have separate rooms for body treatments, complete with chaise-lounge-type chairs without arms that can be adjusted to allow the client to lie perfectly flat. The chair should be covered with clean sheets and soft towels before each individual client. The client should be asked to remove all clothing except underpants and to lie face down on the chair. After covering the body with a sheet or towel, the esthetician then lowers the sheet or towel to just below the waist so that the client's buttocks and legs remain covered, as they are not included in the treatment. (**Fig. 6.1**)

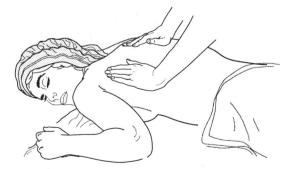

Fig. 6.1. Preparing the client for a back "facial."

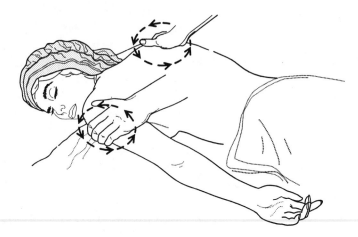

Fig. 6.2. Rotate shoulders, moving fingers to the spine and up to the base of the neck.

A thorough back facial actually starts at the neck and should be geared to the condition of the skin: dry, oily, or blemished. It begins with a gentle cleansing, using a cleansing lotion and warm water on cotton (choose a formula appropriate to the skin type).

For Dry Skin

Start with a light massage. Begin by rotating the shoulders a few times, moving fingers to the spine and then up to the base of the neck. (**Fig. 6.2**) Apply circular movements up to the backs of the ears and then slide fingers to the front of the ears, massaging the upper neck. (**Fig. 6.3**) Gently move down the back, rotating

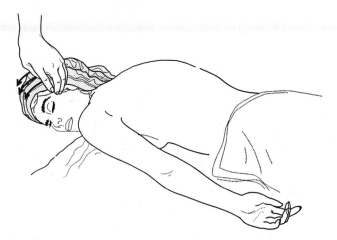

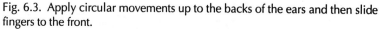

Fig. 6.3. Apply circular movements up to the backs of the ears and then slide fingers to the front.

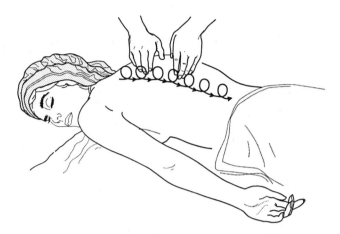

Fig. 6.4. Gently move down the back, rotating fingers in a relaxing circular movement.

the fingers in a relaxing circular motion. (**Fig. 6.4**) The next step is steaming, which should be for about eight minutes maximum for dry skin. To remove the dead cells, a scrub-type mask or a peeling mask should be used (ideally, a gentle scrub mask rubbed into the skin with a soft body brush, then removed with warm water and cotton, is the best choice). As a final touch, a paraffin mask, as described in chapter 4, can then be used, to be removed after ten minutes.

For Oily Skin

When the back is oily, do not do massage, as this could stimulate already overactive oil glands. For the best results, the steaming should last about thirteen minutes. (It's a must to come in and check on clients during steaming to be sure they are not getting too warm or uncomfortable with such a long stretch of steaming. If they are uncomfortable, it's best to cut the steaming time short.) A scrub-type mask should then be used, but without a body brush, and followed up by a pore-cleansing or mud or clay mask as described for use in facials in chapter 3. As a final step, a **seaweed** mask should be applied, left on for twenty minutes, then rinsed off with warm water and cotton, followed by a bracing aloe splash.

For Blemish-Prone Skin

When the skin is blemish-prone, follow the same basic routine as described for oily skin, but omit the scrub mask. If active blemishes are present, substitute a **camphor** mask for the **seaweed** mask in the final step. Follow up with a high-frequency treatment.

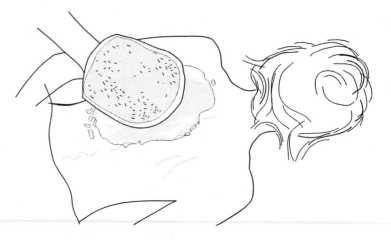

Fig. 6.5. Use a loofah to slough, stimulate, and cleanse.

Because these back treatments are quite gentle on the skin, they can be done as often as once a month, the ideal schedule for those who want to take the best possible care of their body skin. It is also important to counsel your clients on the proper care of their body skin at home, including what type of cleansing routine to follow and the benefits of wearing cool cotton right next to the skin. Hot baths, for example, are wonderful to help dissolve and loosen the skin's impurities, but to really flush away the dirt and dead cells, they should be followed by a brisk shower. Twice a week, a gentle grainy cleanser or acne-type soap should be used on the back, neck, and shoulders, for a deeper clean than soap can give. A **camphor-based drying lotion** should be applied nightly to any skin eruptions. Scrubbing down with a **loofah** is wonderful for sloughing, stimulating, and cleansing but is not a good idea for someone whose back tends to break out. (**Fig. 6.5**)

MASSAGE: THE ULTIMATE IN BODY PAMPERING

For five thousand years, both practitioners and recipients have touted the benefits of "hands-on" massage, which are claimed to range from relieving mental and physical fatigue to improving circulation, general body tone, and the function of muscles and joints. Massage can bring relief from stiff, aching muscles and revitalize tired legs and feet, as well as loosening and relaxing tightness in the neck, shoulders, and lower back. At its best, a one-hour massage can be like a minivacation, leaving a client feeling reenergized and revitalized, able to face the stresses and pressures of everyday life with a new enthusiasm.

Not just anyone can provide a true therapeutic massage, however; it requires training, knowledge, and professional experience. A good massage reflects a combination of anatomical knowledge, personal experience, practical skill, and sensitivity to a client's needs. Yet in some states anyone can hang out a shingle and claim to be a massage expert. That doesn't mean that an esthetician or salon should think lightly about offering massage, however.

In the states of Ohio, New York, Oregon, Washington, Nebraska, and Florida, people must pass comprehensive tests to be granted a license to offer professional massage. Currently, there are licensing requirements of various strictness in about half the states in the United States. There are also fifty-five schools across the country with programs approved by the American Massage Therapy Association (AMTA) Commission on Massage Training Accreditation/Approval. More than ten thousand members of the AMTA have passed written and practical exams in the practice of massage therapy, and AMTA members are required to take continuing education programs every two years. For those specializing in Swedish technique, the Swedish Institute of Massage in New York City is often cited as a strong training center.

These qualifications shouldn't be taken lightly. Massage is a powerful tool, but its powers should be used properly—meaning both in a highly professional manner and in a way that will help ease muscle tensions, not create muscle problems. A poorly given massage can do more than turn clients off to a salon; it can even cause lasting discomfort.

Nowhere is a professional attitude more important than in the segment of a salon devoted to massage (in no way do you want to create the atmosphere of a so-called massage parlor). A salon that offers massage treatments must, first and foremost, be able to provide the space required. It is important not only to have adequately sized massage rooms (there should be ample width for the masseuse to move around the client easily), but also to have shower facilities, so that clients can rinse off any excess creams, oils, or talcs before getting back into their clothes. A comfortable, padded table designed especially for massage is a must, as are plenty of clean sheets, towels, and a small sink and liquid soap for use by the masseuse. All sheets and towels should be changed completely after each client. The

cleanliness of the entire room and salon area cannot be empha-
sized strongly enough; in fact, it is shocking that, in this day of
fears about diseases and infection, massage is still not tightly reg-
ulated in some states. A lack of laws, however, is no excuse for
not taking the care to make your own salon or salon area as
spotless and sanitary as possible.

Because massage is a body treatment, it is crucial that, for
reasons of propriety, clients be asked to remove all their clothes,
except their underwear, in privacy, and then to lie down under
a sheet or extra-large towel. The person giving the massage
should uncover only the area of the body being worked on at
that moment, re-covering each area before proceeding to the

SPOTLIGHT
. . . .
My first experience with a body massage was a funny and intimidating one. I had
never had a stranger touch my body before. But, being in the beauty business, I felt
I had to try it.

When I called to make an appointment at the NYC salon, the receptionist asked
if I would prefer a male or female massage therapist. I decided to jump in head
first and asked for a male practitioner. When I arrived at the salon, I wondered if I
had made a mistake. All kinds of thoughts crossed my mind as I lay on a table in a
dimly lit room in my underwear bottoms. Not knowing massage-room etiquette, I
was lying on my stomach waiting for a good-looking guy to come in and start rubbing me down. The first thing I got, though, was a lecture about the etiquette of
massage and the fact that I should use the large towel to cover my body and turn
over onto my back.

Once the massage started, out of nervousness, I began to make idle chitchat. I
could sense that the masseur knew I was nervous. My body tensed up each time
he touched my shoulder or neck.

Incredibly, once the massage got under way and the relaxation techniques took
hold, the more my stress melted away. I felt the knots in my shoulders, which I
thought were permanent, disappear. The tension in my back gradually became nil.
When he began massaging my feet, that's when I forgot where I was and just felt
totally relaxed.

After the session was over, I felt I had new energy and was able to think more
clearly. I would recommend massage sessions to anyone who suffers from a stressful life—and these days, who doesn't? At a later date, I went on to try a masseuse.
But that's another story.

next, so that the client never feels undressed as the massage progresses. The masseuse or masseur should always wear spotlessly clean clothes, use plenty of deodorant, and be impeccably well groomed. If your unisex salon offers massage, strongly consider offering the option of a male or female massage therapist to clients.

There are numerous types of massage, ranging from traditional **Swedish** massage to **Shiatsu** to "light" massage, pressure-point treatments, hand massage, neck-and-shoulder varieties, and **reflexology**, which focuses on the feet and legs. Some massage specialists prefer to concentrate on one or two types; others offer a variety of options. In a skin care salon, the focus should be on massage as relaxation and pampering, not on treating people after injuries (although some massage practitioners do specialize in sports massage, this is more likely to be offered at a health club or sports medicine facility). It is crucial to ask the client, before beginning any type of massage, if she has high blood pressure (a no-no for heating up the body), any heart problems, or is pregnant (light massage is all right early on, but later in pregnancy it should be avoided). Clients should be advised not to eat immediately before a massage treatment, as it could cause stomach upset.

In a skin care salon setting, the focus should also be on pampering the skin during the massage (although a body massage should never be combined with a facial; these services should be kept properly separate). The hands of the person giving the massage should never directly rub against the client's skin. One of three different types of skin protectors should be used: either **avocado oil**, **talc** (for those prone to back breakouts), or a light massage cream. It is a good idea to ask the client if she or he has a preference before beginning, as some people are allergic to certain ingredients or may not like the feel of oils on the skin. The neck and shoulders are usually part of a massage treatment, but body oils should never be used on the face, because they can clog pores and cause breakouts.

Just as the massage specialist must treat clients in a professional manner, clients should always respect the person giving the massage. Any sexual comments or overtures should lead the practitioner to stop the treatment *immediately* and ask the client to leave, summoning the salon manager if necessary. That client should then be informed that she or he is no longer welcome in the salon. Though it is unusual to focus on turning down potential clients, anyone who violates the professionalism of a salon should no longer be considered a potential client.

WRAPPING IT ALL UP: THE BODY BEAUTIFIERS

Twelve years ago the words **body wraps** were more likely to summon up images of a sarong rather than a luxurious beauty treatment. Within the past five years, all that has changed, as Americans became devotees of spa vacations and were exposed to the kind of pampering treatments that many European women have enjoyed for years. As people started frequenting **spas** and mixing in a dose of relaxation with their exercise regimes, the numbers of clients asking skin care salons about body treatments multiplied. For clients who read about spa vacations but couldn't afford to indulge in them, the local skin care salon became a place they could slip away to for a smaller, but no less luxurious, dose of pampering.

The Seaweed Wrap

The most intensive moisturizing treatments for the body are **body wraps**. One of the most highly prized of these treatments is the **seaweed wrap**, using 100 percent natural marine essences. **Seaweed**, or **algae**, is made of cellular tissue with thick, jelly-like cell walls that contain skin-nourishing proteins. Usually supplied to salons in a concentrated powder form, to be mixed with water into a paste, seaweed masks can help restore skin's elasticity, "rebalance" the skin's water and pH balance, and help strengthen the skin's own cell walls, helping them to conserve moisture. Many marine experts claim that seaweed body masks can help purify, disinfect, and cleanse the skin's functioning.

If these claims sound extreme, that's because they are. Seaweed- and algae-based beauty treatments have come in for a fair amount of criticism from some experts who doubt the ability of this simple substance to have such profound effects. But clients provide all the impetus many salon owners need to offer these treatments: they ask for them, find them incredibly relaxing, and want to come back again for more. Whether or not the treatments do everything that's claimed becomes, in a way, beside the point.

Before considering offering such treatments, there are a few things to keep in mind. Seaweed wraps are definitely messy. You must have a plentiful supply of towels for clients and estheticians both (and the esthetician needs a plentiful supply of uniforms—no one wants to be greeted by someone who has green splotches on her uniform). There must be a shower in the room for clients to rinse thoroughly afterward, plus someone to

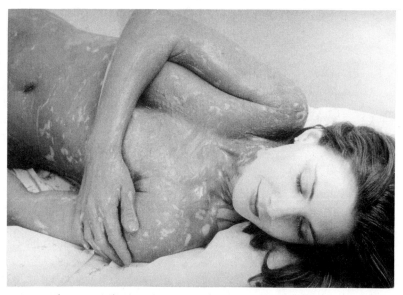

Fig. 6.6. The seaweed wrap. (Courtesy of Steve Victor, M.D.)

clean the shower afterward to be sure it's not coated with greenish mask.

A proper seaweed wrap should begin with a relaxing twenty-five-minute massage. The client then undresses completely. A mix of seaweed powder and warm water (or milk, if skin is extremely dry) is then brushed onto the skin with a soft paint-brush (obviously avoiding the genital and anal areas). (**Fig. 6.6**) The body is then wrapped with thin silver paper (sold through beauty supply houses in long, body-length sheets) and covered with a warm blanket. The client then relaxes for twenty to twenty-five minutes, during which time the esthetician should check that she is still comfortable.

<u>NOTE</u>: Before offering clients this service, be sure to check that they are not allergic to **iodine**, a key ingredient in seaweed powder.

The client is then unwrapped and escorted to a warm shower. A clean robe and towels should be left for her.

The Mud Wrap

Just as the seaweed wrap is ideal for dry skin, the **mud wrap** is the top choice for oily skin, and is especially good for clients with oiliness on the back and chest. Mud masks are made from clays found deep under the sea, which are high in potassium and provide an excellent buffer for the skin, helping the exchange of water between cells and acting as a wonderfully efficient yet gentle cleanser. For clients whose skin is oily, mud is the best type of deep cleanser there can be. Its use as a body treatment basically follows the same steps as previously described for seaweed body wraps. Again, this is a messy but very rewarding treatment. For the esthetician, there is one important caveat, however: not all beauty muds are the same. The best grades of **marine clay** are light gray or brown in the raw, wet state, and turn almost white as they dry (if a clay doesn't lighten as it dries, it's probably not top grade). A high-quality mud will remain in its ready-to-use state for several months if stored in a tightly sealed container; if slight drying occurs, adding a little water should bring it back to its original consistency.

The Paraffin Wrap

The other type of body wrap that is frequently offered is the **paraffin wrap**, which is basically a body-length version of the facial treatment described in chapter 4. Because this type of treatment locks in natural body heat, it is important to be sure ahead of time that a client has no health problems, such as high blood pressure or thyroid troubles, that make exposure to heat unwise.

WHAT'S SO "HOT" ABOUT REFLEXOLOGY AND AROMATHERAPY?

For the past few years, both reflexology and aromatherapy have gotten quite a bit of publicity, with no signs of its stopping. Considered exotic, Eastern-inspired treatments, they are praised for their therapeutic as well as rejuvenating results. A beauty salon practitioner should not concentrate on the alleged health benefits, but the relaxation results might make you or the owner of your salon want to offer these treatments.

Reflexology

An "art of the hands," so to speak, reflexology is based on a principle of Oriental medicine: there are specific parts of the feet that correlate directly with various body parts, and by massaging the feet you can thus relax and free up the body as a whole. One center of knowledge for these types of treatments in the United States is The Reflexology Institute in Florida, which offers hands-on training sessions that can be scheduled at a salon.

Aromatherapy

By using essential oils, ranging from **flowers** to **jojoba** to **almonds**, aromatherapy treats, "heals," and beautifies the skin. These oils are often used in combination with massage to add a potent skin-moisturizing or cleansing effect. After the massage, the aromatherapy oil mixture is worked into the skin using relaxing massage strokes; the body is then wrapped in warm towels and blankets and the client is left to relax for about twenty-five minutes. Then the oils are showered off. A wide variety of companies supply aromatherapy oils to the beauty business. As with any product line, quality varies, as does cost, so be sure to sample specific oils before purchasing large amounts for a salon. Also, inquire about the type of training that is provided along with the product line; some companies have very thorough information programs and others are simply sales organizations with little or no support for salon staff.

Anticellulite Treatment

A final type of body care that draws a lot of attention is **anticellulite treatment**, perhaps one of the most controversial areas for many years now. These body treatments, originated by the French, promise to break down the fatty areas often found around the hips and thighs, which many women claim are totally resistant to diet and exercise. Special creams, body brushes, and sponges and various types of massage methods are often part of these treatments, which may be scheduled two or more times weekly over the course of several weeks. Some creams contain **caffeine**, others **marine algae** or other natural substances claimed to help break down recalcitrant body fat. Devotees of anticellulite treatments claim they get results unmatched by diet or exercise.

Even salon owners who don't completely believe these claims may feel obligated to offer these services, because they don't want to lack anything offered by the competition. Even medical experts who scoff at the long-term claim that massage can eliminate body fat do admit that these massages might have a short-term benefit of seeming to eliminate unwanted bulges, simply by massaging away fluid deposits in the fatty tissue and giving the illusion of slimming the body temporarily. The only problem: If this is the sole benefit, the fluid will come back within a few hours, so the benefits will disappear disappointingly quickly.

SELF-QUIZ: QUESTIONS TO CONSIDER

Massage doesn't seem like such a big deal. We've all given a friend or family member a back rub. Why all the fuss about credentials?

Author's Advice: Like any service, massage should be offered professionally or not at all. After all, we are discussing giving these treatments to strangers and charging money for them. It is only common courtesy to insist that they be worthwhile relaxation treatments rather than casual rubdowns. Also, a poorly done massage can cause muscle strain or injury at worst, and muscle discomfort at the least, all of which reflects badly on the salon as a whole and could lose you customers.

I have heard that some customers feel claustrophobic when getting body wraps. How common is this?

Author's Advice: There are no exact statistics to say how common this reaction is, but it does exist. That is why it is important to ascertain, before leaving the room, whether the client is comfortable and to explain to clients how long they will be wrapped. It is also crucial to come back in after a few minutes to see that the client feels comfortable—not too hot or too closed-in—and to recheck at least several times during a twenty-minute session.

I have seen promises of real health benefits from aroma-therapy treatments. Are these true?

Author's Advice: In Europe, aromatherapy is used in many medical clinics as an adjunct to other treatments. In this country, however, the federal government has not approved any such claims, and it would be unwise (as well as illegal) for a beauty salon to advertise or promote anything of a health-oriented nature; this could be construed as practicing medicine without a license.

The purpose of aromatherapy treatments in a skin care salon should be to promote relaxation and the resulting skin benefits. Certain preparations are available that claim to encourage smooth skin, decrease oiliness or dryness, and improve overall circulation, which is important to the skin's appearance. These are the uses best suited to a skin care salon's services.

CHAPTER 7   Hair Removal Treatments

In Europe, it is not uncommon for teenage girls to be brought to beauty salons by their mothers to discuss the question of unwanted hair; in America, surprisingly, the whole topic is still somewhat of a taboo subject. The reason, more than anything else, is misunderstanding of the fact that unwanted hair is not necessarily abnormal hair. Although so-called excess hair is often a source of embarrassment and lowered self-esteem—for men as well as women—hair growth is a perfectly normal body function. Hormonal problems are sometimes responsible for the sudden appearance of unwanted facial or body hair, but in the majority of cases what brings on unhappiness about hair growth is the simple fact that, compared to the plucked, shaved, and waxed perfection of models in the pages of glossy magazines, everyone seems to have too much body hair. In this chapter, you will learn about:

- when to treat or not treat excess hair
- who needs professional hair-removal treatments
- basic procedures for waxing, electrolysis, and tweezing
- how to advise clients about bleaching and use of hair-removal creams
- hair-removal services for men: should you offer them?

THE NOT-SO-BARE FACTS

Considering that the average person's face has more than 25,000 hair follicles on its surface, it's not surprising that some of them seem to grow where and when they're not wanted. According to dermatologists, more than 85 percent of women have hair on their arms and legs—although you'd never know it from the artificially smoothed surfaces of cover models and actresses (whose skin, if it isn't already perfect, is frequently air-brushed to unnatural smoothness in photographs by the art directors of top magazines).

There are basically two different kinds of hair that grow on the human body. **Vellus** hair is fine, short, and almost colorless; it is the so-called baby hair that's found just about everywhere on the body (the only places it can't grow are on the palms of one's hands and the soles of one's feet). **Terminal** hair is thicker, pigmented, and very visible; at puberty, when androgens (male hormones) are produced by the body, some areas of vellus hair begin to convert to terminal hair. In women, the amount of body hair that becomes visible depends on genetics to a large part; if a woman's mother, siblings, and aunts all had excess hair, chances are she will too. Those with dark hair and dark complexions often have more visible body hair than those who are fair skinned and light haired.

True excess hair, or **hirsutism**, occurs when women develop an overabundance of hair in a male pattern on the upper lip, chin, sides of the cheeks, chest, abdomen, and thighs. If the hair in this area is thick and long, the client should probably be checked by a physician who can rule out such possible causes as an over- or underactive thyroid gland, adrenal gland imbalances, multiple sclerosis, diabetes, or the side effects of drugs used to treat conditions such as high blood pressure, mood disorders, or fibrocystic breast disease. In some cases, dermatologists do treat excess hair growth that is not associated with a specific medical problem with antiandrogen medications. The theory is that because the hair has become overresponsive to the natural level of these male hormones within a woman's body, a medication that blocks these hormones can block the excess hair growth. The problem, however, is that these drugs may have side effects ranging from lowered sex drive to dry and itching skin, nausea, depression, fatigue, rises in blood pressure, and liver problems. Steroid-type medicines are sometimes used, but these also can have serious side effects.

Just as puberty's hormonal changes can give rise to unwanted hair growth, so can the hormonal upsurges that occur with pregnancy or menopause. As women age, it's not uncommon for a few bristle-like hairs to develop on the chin or upper lip. Because these are permanent and often isolated, they are commonly treated with minor **electrolysis**.

THE PROFESSIONAL ADVANTAGE: SALON SERVICES

In general, beauty salons offer three methods of hair removal:
1.   waxing (of face and body)
2.   tweezing (of eyebrows)

3.   electrolysis—the only permanent method (used primarily for face but also, less commonly, for body)

Shaving, bleaching, and hair-removal creams are used by many women at home; advising them on the best procedures to follow is also a good undertaking for skin care salons.

Waxing: Not All Methods Are the same

Waxing is a common beauty-salon hair-removal method because it removes hair close to the root, providing a smooth result that keeps the area free of hair for three to six weeks, depending on the thickness of a client's hair growth. There are two types of wax: hard wax and the softer strip method (cold-wax treatments, although sold for home use, do not provide the kind of quality results required in a salon). Some practitioners use the same type of wax for face and body areas, but experience shows that they do not provide the same consistent results. **Hard wax** is best used on facial areas—above the lips, on the chin, and between the brows; **strip wax** provides much better results on arms, legs, and the bikini area. Although some skin care salons use wax on larger facial areas, waxing the cheeks is a very unsatisfactory choice, because regrowth is immediately—and unattractively—apparent.

Waxing is very technique dependent; approximately 20 percent of the clients who come to my salon say that they have had a bad experience with waxing at a salon in the past. Gentleness is key in terms of the wax temperature, application, and post-waxing skin care. No educational requirements are mandated by the states for this type of hair-removal treatment, but experience should be the greatest teacher. It's important for all estheticians to learn from clients' less-than-perfect experiences, too. Every first-time client should be asked about any past waxings (whether the skin reacted, etc.) before beginning.

FACIAL WAXING should be done in a facial treatment room that is clean and prepared ahead of time. The wax should be melted in an automatic melting machine made just for that purpose. The setting should be put on low and fresh wax must be used with every single client.

Waxing must be done on a clean skin surface. A small towel should be wrapped around the client's neck and the hair covered; then the skin should be cleansed of all makeup. Wet cotton pads should be placed over the eyes. A special powder recommended for waxing should then be applied to the skin.

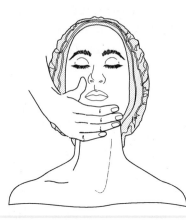

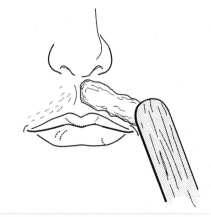

Fig. 7.1. The skin may burn after pulling off the wax; to help soothe the area, simply press your palms against the skin.

Fig. 7.2. Apply wax using a spatula.

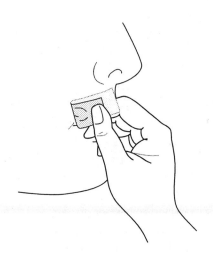

Fig. 7.3. Muslin should be pulled up in a matter of seconds.

Take a tiny bit of wax on a fresh cotton swab and check the temperature on the inside of your wrist. If the wax is not too hot, apply thin layers of wax to the facial areas to be treated. Leave the wax on for one minute—literally, no longer—and then pull it off against the direction that the hair naturally grows. To lessen the stinging that naturally occurs, follow immediately with pressure from the palm of your hand on the skin. (**Fig. 7.1**) A cool compress or calamine or seaweed mask can be used to take any redness away; in no case should a customer leave your salon with red blotches on the skin.

NOTE: In the above-the-lip area, apply the wax from the center outward in two separate pieces, as the hair grows in two different directions. (**Figs. 7.2, 7.3**)

BODY WAXING is best done using strip wax that is removed using **muslin fabric strips**. The muslin can be bought in a roll and cut in the salon, or bought pre-cut to the size of about six inches by two inches (of course, pre-cut strips are much more costly). New wax must be used with every client; under no circumstances should wax be reused! This includes the use of machines that supposedly filter out hair to allow reuse of wax. In an age when disease prevention is a key interest, and sanitary methods of sterilizing everything in the salon are recommended, there is no excuse for reusing hair-removal wax. As additional precautions, wax should never be stored around heat (it can go bad) and should never be left in a heating machine for too long. About an hour before a client is booked for a waxing session, the wax should be melted; any wax that remains should be discarded immediately afterward, and the pot should be cleaned.

As with the face, wax should be applied to a clean skin surface; a gentle toner can be used if the skin is oily or very heavy body lotion has been used. Using a fresh wooden spatula, changed for each client, apply a small amount of wax to an area of the skin. Immediately apply a muslin fabric strip over the wax and pull it right up in a matter of seconds. Check to see whether any reaction occurs and do not proceed if the client seems overly sensitive. (**Fig. 7.4**) Consider trying again with slightly cooler wax or advise against having waxing at this time.

Assuming no reaction occurs, proceed with the waxing by treating small areas (roughly two inches by four inches) at a time, applying the wax in the direction of hair growth with the spatula

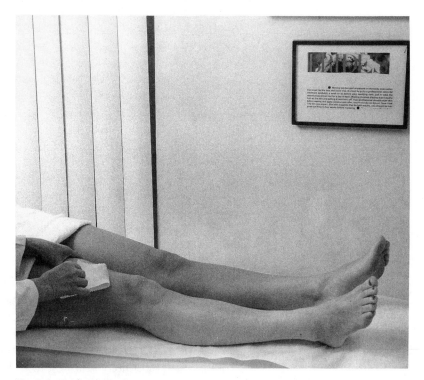

Fig. 7.4. Body waxing.

held at a 45-degree angle to the skin, smoothing the fabric strip over in the same direction, and leaving an edge free. Grasp the fabric with one hand, using the other hand to keep the skin taut, and pull the fabric in the opposite direction of the hair growth. If the wax comes right off the muslin strip, the strip itself can be reused once or twice. What is key is working in small areas. If you wait to do half a leg before removing the wax, it will be hardened by the time you pull it off and the skin will inevitably be irritated. The prime reason that so many clients find waxing painful or irritating is that the wax is simply left on too long. It doesn't take very long to bond with the hair, but the longer it's left on, the more it also bonds to the skin, causing irritation and blotchiness once it is pulled off. It is also crucial to check on the wax temperature, to be sure that it is warm but not hot.

Waxing in the Bikini Area   The bikini area is the most sensitive area of the body and attention must be paid to avoiding irritation. Ideally, bikini waxing should be done every two and a half to three weeks throughout the year; over time, it can then be done much less frequently, as the hair becomes much weaker and grows much more slowly. If the hair is very long, and a client has never had a bikini wax before, the hair should be cut with scrupulously sterilized scissors. A patch test should be done, treating a one-inch area of the uppermost thigh, to be sure that the client is not allergic to the wax, or that the skin does not overreact (although some skin sensitivity is not uncommon the first few times, it should not be severe).

Ask the customer how far up she wants the waxing to go, but also use your own careful judgment; the mucous membranes of the vagina are hypersensitive, and the last thing you want to cause is vaginal irritation. Warn new clients that waxing is always painful the first few times it is done, especially in this area. _Never_ use oil-based creams or lotions on this skin area; soothe the skin afterward with an oatmeal-based powder, which is gentler even than talc. Sometimes bumps or ingrown hairs develop in the bikini area; isolated hairs can be removed via tweezing or electrolysis.

Although most clients think of bikini waxing as something that needs to be done in the summer only, or if they're headed for a midwinter tropical vacation, the best results are achieved by continuing to wax all year round, because the hair weakens over time and then waxings can become less frequent, and also much less potentially irritating to the skin. At many salons, discount packages for six or ten waxing sessions are offered to encourage clients to come regularly. Of course, if a client prefers not to, then you still try to give them the best possible results when they do come later on.

Another key to a professional result is to leave the skin smooth, not sticky. After the waxing is completed, take clean fabric strips and go over the skin to remove any stray wax. **(Fig. 7.5)** There are four preferred choices of what to use on the skin to soothe and prevent redness:

1. aloe gel for very sensitive skin

2. talc for sensitive skin

3. an astringent diluted with a little water for skin that's not overly sensitive

4. astringent mixed with a few drops of body oil for thicker skin.

Whatever you choose, be sure the skin is not blotchy or irritated when the client leaves the salon. Don't neglect to use your common sense: successful waxing depends on the hair being long enough to bond to the wax. Many women have come to my salon requesting underarm waxing before a special vacation—after they have already tried to get the area perfectly smooth via shaving. My response to them is that trying to wax then would only produce irritation. Although waxing can be

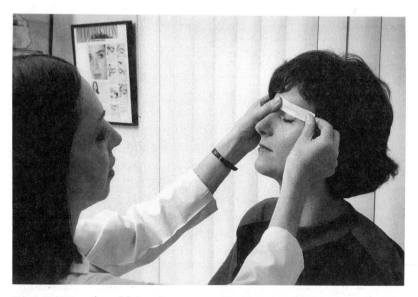

Fig. 7.5. Using clean fabric strips, go over the skin to remove stray wax.

SPOTLIGHT
••••••••••••••••

During the first year of my employment in the United States, I was lucky enough to land a job at a top New York City salon. I was very willing to learn about all of the treatments offered there, but usually wasn't called upon to do anything I hadn't perfected. Until, that is, a client booked for a facial decided that she also wanted her eyebrows waxed—and I was the only one available on such short notice. I told the manager that I really didn't know how to do waxing, but she insisted she would tell me how. That she did, in about two minutes. The result: I applied so much wax that I almost took the woman's eyebrows off completely! Quick reflexes saved her—and my job.

The experience taught me an all-important lesson, though. Something may seem easy, but we all need training to do our jobs correctly. We need to apprentice ourselves to those whose years of practice have helped them perfect the services offered in skin care salons. You need to practice on yourself, your colleagues, and fellow students. And always pay attention to what you are doing, so that any potential disasters can be corrected before harm to a client occurs.

done under the arms, the hair must have been allowed to grow for two weeks. Even then, it must be done in three very small areas under each arm, because the skin there is so fragile and highly prone to irritation. Applying the wax to a very small area and then removing it immediately usually keeps redness to a minimum.

Tweezing: Perfect Brow Shaping

One of the oldest methods of hair removal, **tweezing** is still a good choice when removing just a few stray hairs from around the brows. Many estheticians prefer tweezing to waxing when a woman wants a more natural, bushier-looking brow line, and leave waxing for those who desire a more shaped look.

First-time customers should be thoroughly consulted about the brow shape they want. Don't be abrupt; let the client hold the mirror while you discuss with her how much or how little hair she wants removed, where she wants the curve to be, and whether she wants to maintain or change her natural brow shape. In general, you can encourage a client one way or the other, but you must leave the final decision up to her.

All tweezers used in a salon must be sterilized before and after each use. The brow area should be cleansed with makeup remover to get rid of any brow color or eye shadow that extends up to the brow area. Follow with a gentle cleansing solution and then use your fingers to press the brow upwards so the actual plucking isn't felt as much. Although tweezer styles are a matter of personal choice, the type with an **angled bottom** is usually easier to manipulate than those with a **v-shaped** point or **flat edge**. If in doubt about how much to tweeze, do less. You can always remove more hairs once the woman has looked at the results, but it will take a good amount of time for hairs to grow back. As women age, their brows naturally get thinner, so less tweezing may be needed. As for brow coloring, it's not uncommon for women to dye their brows once a month if they already use hair coloring. This doesn't really change the need for proper shaping, however.

The perfect post-tweezing treatment is a mild but soothing astringent patted—not rubbed—onto the skin. If a client is overly sensitive and very red, cool compresses may also be used.

Electrolysis: A Permanent but Not Instant Solution

In 1916, the multiple-needle machine was developed and electrolysis came into being. It wasn't until after World War II, however, that the short-wave method was developed, making electrolysis much faster and more effective, producing a truly permanent method of getting rid of unwanted hair. Today, electrolysis is often vaunted as the perfect solution to an embarrassing problem, but even more than other methods, its success depends on the proper technique. The numbers of women who have been scarred by improper electrolysis procedures is really shocking.

The idea of offering electrolysis in a skin care salon seems a natural fit. After all, smooth skin is the goal of estheticians. No one looks more closely at the skin than people in the beauty business. But electrolysis is a specific skill that requires enormous patience and care. The first requirement is that the operator have a **certificate of licensing** in electrolysis in a given state. The second unwritten requirement is that a good electrologist should be highly trained in skin care, so that the skin can be protected from damage during the treatment. Unfortunately, this isn't always the case. Skin can be irritated, capillaries can be damaged, and scar tissue can develop after electrolysis is carelessly performed, either by treating a given follicle too vigorously or treating too many follicles at the same session. Electrolysis is a time-consuming, costly process—and

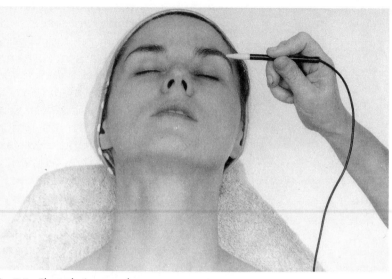

Fig. 7.6. Electrolysis on eyebrows.

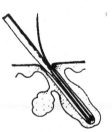

Fig. 7.7. Electrolysis is permanent, literally destroying the hair root via an electric current through the needle.

if that fact is not clear to both the operator and the client, then dangerous rushing of the treatment can occur.

Many proponents of electrolysis claim that it can be used anywhere on the body. It is true that the lips, breasts, and bikini area can be treated without pain if done skillfully; however, hair inside the ears should *never* be removed, nor should any hair growing out of a freckle or mole. Although electrolysis is permanent, literally destroying the root of the hair via an electric current, it is anything but instant. **(Figs. 7.6, 7.7)**

In general, electrolysis takes between six months to two years to fully rid an area of the face or body of all unwanted hair. (Of course, a man who is coming for treatment of just a few ingrown hairs will require fewer visits.) A professional should never promise a client results in a specific amount of time, as it is really impossible to predict with certainty how the hair's cycle will go. It takes from eight to thirteen weeks for a hair to grow up past the surface of the skin, on the average, but it may take longer if the client has been regularly waxing or tweezing. Some clients with heavier hair growth should come once a week at first; others can come less often. It's important to advise waiting until at least six treatments have been completed to start evaluating the success.

Especially in a skin care salon, attention should be paid to protecting the skin from any damage. An antiseptic soothing lotion should always be applied after treatments to prevent infection and soothe skin. Advise clients that if a scab forms, it should *not* be picked off, as this will only increase the chances of infection. Letting the tiny scab heal itself usually means that it will disappear invisibly. Emphasize that there should be no tweezing or waxing of hair at home during the treatment—and no picking on the skin. No makeup should be applied for at least one half hour after an electrolysis treatment. Regrowth will vary, but should not be more than 20 to 25 percent in an area after an initial treatment. Of course, this is not literally regrowth of the follicles that were treated, but activation of follicles that were in the dormant stage. Taking the time to explain all of these points to the client may seem tedious, but it is crucial to the success of the treatment—and the likelihood that a client will want to continue.

Few salons need to employ a full staff of electrologists. It's possible to start with a part-time person, then work up to several days a week, increasing the time as business develops. (Anyone performing electrolysis knows that it is intensive work and requires keen vision. A yearly eye exam is a must.) The machinery used must be approved by the Federal Communications Commission (FCC) and maintained properly; this is no place to skimp on cost and buy an old machine. Some electrologists prefer the older type of short-wave needle machine, while many others advocate the insulated bulbous probe, claiming it is a little less painful and faster to use.

Whatever the type of machine, sterilization is a major issue today in any treatment involving needles. There is really only one fail-safe solution: Have each electrolysis client purchase a needle and bring it with her or him each time, at which time it should be sterilized in the machine. The average cost of a needle is $8 to $15, and the needle will last quite a long time; at worst, it may have to be replaced once or twice.

AT-HOME CONCERNS: SHAVING, BLEACHING, DEPILATORY CREAMS

Not every client will choose to come to a salon for hair-removal treatments, but that doesn't mean the esthetician won't be called on to offer advice on home treatments, especially for women who are regular customers for facials or body wraps. Knowing what to advise is key—and you may even be able to convert a customer to a professional solution after a while.

Shaving: For Men Only?

In most skin care professionals' opinions, shaving should really be left to men to remove their beards, and to women to use under their arms, not on their legs and bikini areas. The reason is that too many women shave carelessly, cutting themselves and using a razor blade so many times that it irritates the skin. Shaving also makes hair stronger and coarser, with the result that one ends up needing to shave the legs more and more often.

If a woman insists on shaving, she should do what a man does: prepare the skin first, by showering and coating the skin with a pre-shave product rich in emollients. She should take care to shave against the direction of hair growth and not to go over an area too many times. Afterward, she should apply a soothing lotion or cream containing **aloe** or **allantoin**.

Bleaching: Beware of Irritation

Faces, lips, and arms are common places to use bleach. Of course, it should always be of the type intended for use on facial hair, but even this can be irritating. **Peroxide** is needed to thoroughly lighten hair and this can be drying, particularly for sensitive complexions. Few, if any, skin care salons offer bleaching, because they are not hair salons. In any case, the aim is not to have less hair but lighter-toned, somewhat less obvious hair.

Bleaching must be done regularly to be effective. Even a slight growth of hair above the lip, for example, can produce an unwelcome shadow. To avoid irritation, never leave bleach on the hair longer than five minutes or so; although some products advise ten minutes, it's not uncommon to get a stinging sensation after that amount of time. Better to treat the hair again for another few minutes later that day, protecting the skin from irritation. Tell clients to be sure to rinse off all bleach solution or cream with cool (never hot) water and to apply a moisturizer immediately afterwards.

Depilatories: Use with Caution

Because they remove hair at the skin surface, so-called hair removal creams are very popular with some clients. The problem from a skin care point of view is that they are very caustic, and because hair and the outermost layer of the epidermis are made of very similar proteins, depilatory creams can damage skin while chemically dissolving away hair. In fact, depilatories are a very common cause of contact **dermatitis**, evidenced by red bumps, most often on thighs or around the bikini area.

Depilatories are available in cream, lotion, spray, and foam forms. Many have new scented varieties to mask the unpleasant odor of the chemicals. The scent ingredients themselves, though, can also cause skin reactions. For that reason, it's vital that clients **patch-test** the product before use, applying it to a very small area of skin, rinsing it off in ten minutes, and then waiting twenty-four hours to see if a reaction occurs.

There are two keys to avoiding any further problems with depilatories:

1. Urge your clients to use a timer and *never* to leave the product on the skin for longer than advised (in fact, it's best to err on the safe side by using it for the minimum specified time).

2. Emphasize that depilatories really should not be used on facial skin, but if they insist, a product specifically formulated for facial use must be used.

SELF-QUIZ: QUESTIONS TO CONSIDER

A long-time client in the salon where I am employed has come for monthly waxings for the past ten years. She thinks her hair is growing more slowly now, and she has asked about coming less often. Is slower hair growth more likely?

Author's Advice: Yes, for two reasons. One is that as we age, hair growth may slow, especially on the legs. In a woman's twenties and thirties, she may need to have her legs waxed once a month to keep them smooth; in her forties, that may stretch to every six weeks or so. Another contributing factor is the effect of regular waxing: over time, it can deaden the hair follicles, almost destroying them or putting them on a slower growth cycle.

If this woman is truly a loyal customer of the salon, give her the respect she deserves. Arrange to have her appointments booked less frequently. Chances are she'll reward the salon's honesty with greater purchases in the long run.

Should every skin care salon offer electrolysis?

Author's Advice: Not necessarily. Electrolysis is a highly specialized skill. A practitioner must not only be licensed by the state, but also should be adept at recognizing the skin's needs and referring any potential medical problems to a dermatologist or endocrinologist. A salon can decide whether to offer this service based on both customer demand and space and commitment to the service.

If your salon does not choose to offer electrolysis on-site, you can easily offer referrals to qualified electrologists in the area by familiarizing yourself with their practices through visits to their offices. A referral to a good solo practitioner will be much appreciated by one's clients.

Some salons have special wax-filtering machines that are claimed to remove all hair and make old wax "good as new." Is this possible?

Author's Advice: Definitely not. The only wax that is as sanitary and safe to use as new wax is truly new wax that has never been used before. The amount of money that can be saved by such practices is dwarfed by the prospect of spreading infection, bacteria, and dirt. A true professional would never use "recycled" wax, regardless of the claims made by manufacturers of filtering machines.

CHAPTER 8

Attracting and Serving the Male Client

Until recent years, it was assumed that skin care services were for women only. Men had skin—and skin problems—but it was perceived as unmanly to care too much about their appearance. "A shave and a haircut," as the old ditty went, was all that a man was supposed to need.

Over the last two decades, though, and especially the last ten years, ideas changed. Men began working out at the gym, not just working their ways up the corporate ladder; they began wearing custom-tailored suits and shopping around for shave creams rather than just buying what the local drugstore had to offer. In the boom years that were the 1980s, the money being spent by men on the care and maintenance of their appearance increased enormously, and the skin care industry was a major beneficiary of that spending.

Today, few skin care salons in major cities are complete without offering services for men as well as women. A few can even claim to have numbers of male clients equal to or greater than their female clients. For that reason, the best estheticians today need to know as much about treating a man's skin as a woman's. Although many of the treatments are very much the same, there are important differences. In this chapter, you will learn about:

- how to talk to a man about his skin and which questions to ask in addition to those you would pose to a woman

- how the salon's environment influences a man's perception of the process of skin care

- the importance of shaving to the condition of a man's skin, and how a good esthetician can help improve the whole process

- ways to build the male clientele in a salon.

CONSULTATION CUES: QUESTIONS NOT TO SKIP

As a general rule, the same attitude that you take toward women clients—caring, supportive, and informative—is the right approach to take with men clients, but with one important difference: men usually need more support for the idea of skin care than do women, especially in their first visits to a salon. After all, men didn't grow up watching their fathers take care of their complexions in the way that little girls observe their mothers applying makeup and moisturizers. Even if a man has actually gone through with making a first appointment at a salon, he still may question the whole value of skin care and wonder whether the idea is a foolish one; after all, his wife or girlfriend may have urged him to visit the salon or given him a gift certificate to come. How the staff treats him and the first impressions he gets are of utmost importance in determining whether he will follow through with a skin care regimen or ever visit the salon again.

Within the past few years, certain trends have helped to make more men comfortable with the idea of skin care. Magazine articles and books discussing the subject, lectures on skin care at health clubs and spas that attract a male clientele, and the advertising of men's skin care products by major cosmetic companies all have opened up the subject to a wider audience. Still, the average man is likely to shy away from the notion of spending a lot of time or energy on taking care of his skin. It's the esthetician's job to make it streamlined and easy for him.

During the first visit or consultation, there are certain key questions to ask. These include:

- **Have you ever had a facial before?** If the client has not, be sure to explain each step as you go along, as straightforwardly as possible. Whereas some women still come to cosmetics counters and skin care salons expecting miracles in a jar, most men do not.

- **How did you hear about the salon?** If the client is there at the urging of someone who is already a regular at the salon, you will have the benefit of convincing evidence. A man who has seen an improvement in his wife's, girlfriend's, or friend's skin is likely to be a little less skeptical than someone who hasn't seen firsthand what skin care experts can do.

- **How often do you shave?** Some men with especially heavy beards shave twice a day, once in the morning before work and again before going out at night; others with light beards may shave every other day or even every third day. Frequent shavers may think they are most prone to skin problems from shaving, but that is not necessarily the case. It's how a man prepares his skin before shaving that matters most to the condition of his skin.

- **Do you have any skin problems?** Along with shaving problems, breakouts are a key reason many men come to skin care salons. Oily skin is often the starting point, but stress can exacerbate the problem. Wrinkles and sun damage may also be a motivating factor, as can the tired look that comes from too much stress.

- **Have you ever had allergic reactions to any skin care products?** Because men do shave and exfoliate their skin on an everyday basis, male skin can sometimes be more sensitive to fragrances or other potential skin irritants or allergens. It's important to ask ahead of time if a man has had rashes, stinging, or itchiness that could be traced to a particular kind of product or ingredient, so that you can avoid as many bad reactions as possible.

As with female clients, it's important to fill out a **consultation card** or record when you see a male client for the first time. On this card or paper you should record details about the appearance of the skin: whether it's dry, dehydrated, sensitive, or oily; whether it has open pores, **comedones** (blackheads), **milia** (whiteheads), or more severe acne breakouts; whether there are scars, wrinkles, deep lines, or discolorations. (**Fig. 8.1**) A

CONSULTATION CARD

Name_____ Date of Consultation _____

Address _____ Age _____ Sex_____

City _____ State _____ Zip_____ Known allergies_____

Tel. (Home) _____ (Business) _____ _____

Ref. by:_____ Medication_____
        (Person, advertising, etc)   _____

SKIN CLASSIFICATION

Facial Area	Facial Area

Normal_____ Acne _____How many years_____

Dry_____   Vulgaris _____Chronic_____

Dehydrated _____   Cystic _____Rosacea_____

Aging _____ Scars (acne, etc.)_____

Thin, sensitive skin_____ Wrinkles_____

Oily _____ Good elasticity _____

Open pores _____ Broken capillaries _____

Comedones (blackheads) _____ Discolorations_____

Milium (whiteheads) _____

REMARKS_____

_____

_____

_____

Rec. Treatment_____

_____

Fig. 8.1. The consultation card.

difference in men's skin here is that many men have two different kinds of skin: one in the area where they shave and one where they don't. Many men have soft, almost baby-like skin in the areas that are shaved every day, thanks to the benefits of **exfoliation**; others who are especially sensitive or use misguided shaving techniques may have highly irritated skin where they shave. The neck is often a very sensitive skin area for men, because of shaving, whereas women's eye area is more likely to show irritation due to daily makeup application and removal.

THE SALON SETTING: BEWARE OF RIBBONS AND LACE

Despite the fact that more men than ever before visit skin care salons, there is still a good deal of trepidation among many men. In fact, some men actually seem to approach coming for their first facial as a challenge—not to themselves but to the esthetician; their attitude is almost one of daring the facialist to prove that she knows what she's talking about! Others still harbor the gut feeling that a skin care center is a place for women only—a reaction that unfortunately can be borne out by the decor and room arrangements in some skin care establishments.

A skin care center is a place of service to its clients; it should look clean, neat, and welcoming. If a salon is geared to both male and female clients, it should not have a waiting room filled with lacy, beribboned pillows that are reminiscent of a woman's boudoir. This isn't to suggest that there can't be feminizing touches, such as pastel flowers or soft colors, but some effort should be made to accommodate the actual skin care clientele. If that clientele includes—or you want it to include—a healthy percentage of men, then the atmosphere should be as androgynous as possible. (**Fig. 8.2**) This includes not just the overall decor but also the details. Magazines in the waiting area, for example, shouldn't cater exclusively to female readers. (Of course, this applies to any salon; even an exclusively female clientele might appreciate being able to peruse a news magazine as well as a fashion publication.) Robes and towels used during facials should be in neutral tones (actually, white is the generally preferred color, because of its fresh, clean impression, regardless of the clients' gender). Publicity materials or articles displayed in the salon should deal with caring for men's skin as well as women's.

The question often arises as to whether a skin care center should have a separate men's area. The answer depends on knowing the clients and the culture in that particular city or

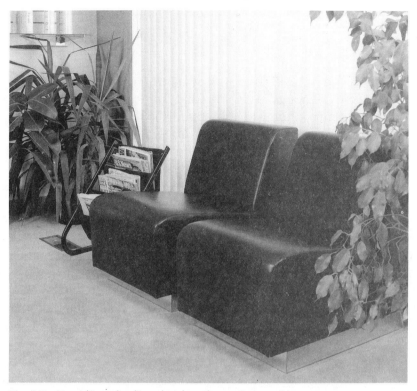

Fig. 8.2. Consider male clientele when decorating a waiting room.

area of the country. For example, a skin care center in the South might do better to have a separate men's waiting room as well as treatment rooms, whereas a Los Angeles salon might find this totally unnecessary. In areas in which space is somewhat limited, a compromise could be made. One or two treatment rooms could be designated for men only, in which a male client could not only have his facial but could also have a manicure in privacy, rather than in an open nail-treatment area, should he so prefer. Other factors that can make men more comfortable in a salon are to have some male employees, such as the salon manager or assistants (if not estheticians), so that the staff doesn't add to the incorrect impression that this is a woman-only environment. Another alternative used by many salons is to have special men's days, during which the salon is primarily geared to offering services to men or even, in some places, days on which women literally can't get appointments. In that way, the hesitant male client doesn't feel as if he is the only man at a women's salon.

SPOTLIGHT
••••••••••••••••••

During the early 1970s, I worked at the famous Georgette Klinger salon on Madison Avenue in New York City. This was the first skin care salon to open its doors to men, and I was chosen, in what I now consider a lucky accident, to head up the men's salon. Ms. Klinger, in her usual way, was prescient: I had no idea (but she seemed to) that I would be good at making men feel interested about and comfortable with the whole idea of skin care.

We had the same entrance as the main salon, but a separate waiting area and separate treatment rooms. The first thing I learned was that although the men who booked appointments had made the first brave step toward caring for their skin, they were often intimidated and uncertain about the "whole skin thing," as former President George Bush might have put it. Their questions ranged along the same lines as women's, but their base of knowledge was often much narrower. What they knew about skin creams and cleansers was what they'd learned by looking in their mothers', wives', or girlfriends' section of the medicine cabinet—men's magazines didn't write very much about taking care of a man's skin in those days!

When I left Georgette Klinger to start my own salon in the early 1980s, I was firmly committed to providing the best possible skin care to both women and men. It was the right time in our society: men were focusing on dressing right and looking right and were willing to invest money in their appearance. I also found that the press, whether in newspapers or magazines, was hungry for information about skin troubles and how to clear them up, for both the men and the women in their readership. Television shows even invited me as a guest to focus specifically on men's skin care. One friend of a friend woke up in London one morning while on a business trip, turned on the news, and was surprised to hear me discussing the "science of shaving" while he was performing his morning ritual with shaving cream and razor.

Today, my clientele is made up of as many men as women. The biggest change I've seen is that while in the 1970s it was embarrassing for many men to set foot anywhere near a skin care salon, in the 1990s taking care of oneself is recognized as a key factor in having a long, healthy life.

SHAVING: THE KEY TO A MAN'S SKIN CONDITION

Shaving is the one skin care routine that most men follow, beginning in their teens. But it's also a process that can either mar the skin, through repeated nicks and cuts, or keep it smooth and young-looking, if the proper techniques are used.

Few men think much about the process of shaving. To them it's a necessity, often done automatically, much like brushing one's teeth. An esthetician can usually tell from her first look at a man's skin under the magnifying lens whether he is shaving correctly—setting up the hairs and his skin for the coming assault and soothing the newly exposed skin afterwards—or whether he's attacking the hairs on his face along with his complexion. A good esthetician usually can help almost every man improve his technique.

Shaving not only removes unwanted hairs from the face, it also lifts off dead skin cells, encouraging the exfoliation that is the key to smoother, younger-looking skin. What we think of as healthy skin is translucent, even-surfaced, and readily reflects light. Shaving, when done correctly, helps keep skin free of the debris that can dull its appearance. But done too roughly, this same exfoliation can cause excessive skin dryness and irritation, removing skin cells that are not ready to be removed, or aggravating already flaky skin conditions.

To help a man get the best shave possible, in terms of removing the hair and protecting the skin, there are certain questions a facialist can ask:

- **How long does it usually take you to shave your face?** Any answer of less than five minutes is a red flag. Rushing is often the culprit in shaving "battle scars."

- **What type of razor do you use?** The choice between a **straight razor** and an **electric** one is a matter of personal preference, but whichever a man uses, he should always use pre- and post-shave products formulated for that specific method. The equipment—meaning the shaver itself and the man's hands—should always be clean and fresh.

- **Do you shave with or against your hair's natural growth direction?** If a man can't answer this, and his skin looks razor-burnt, you've found a problem shaver. Whether a man chooses to shave with or against the natural hair growth pattern is a matter of personal choice, but the important point is to adopt one method and try to stick with it to avoid going over a skin area in different directions—a sure route to skin irritation. (**Fig. 8.3**) On the neck, the hair often grows in several different directions. A man with this pattern can shave in different directions as long as he doesn't go over the same area more than twice.

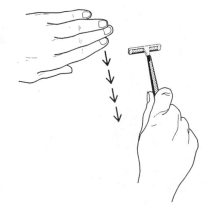

Fig. 8.3. Shave in one direction only.

- **How do you prepare your face before shaving?** If a man uses a **straight razor**, he should cleanse his face first, preferably using a cleansing lotion rather than soap. He should then splash lots of warm water on his face to soften the beard and help "open" the pores (alternatively, shaving after a shower or bath is ideal, especially if skin is sensitive). A gentle wash-off cream or moisturizer (sometimes called a pre-shave) should be applied to the skin, followed by a shaving cream, foam, or gel. (**Fig. 8.4**) Then the man should wait for two minutes to "set up" his beard before beginning to shave.

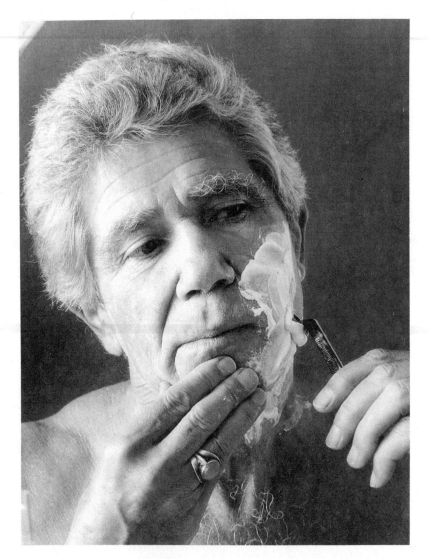

Fig. 8.4. Be sure to properly prepare the skin with a moisture-rich shaving cream.

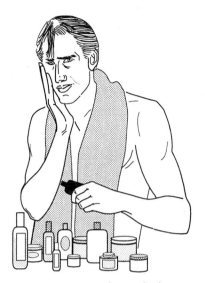

Fig. 8.5. Suggest and provide shaving products.

A problem many men have is that they do everything in a big rush—splash the face, apply a dab of shaving cream, and immediately start to shave—and end up getting lots of nicks and cuts.

A man who uses an **electric razor** has to be sure that his skin is as dry as possible before shaving. For this reason, it's important to wait a little while (a minute or so) between washing one's face and shaving, and then to apply a pre-shave product designed for use with electric shavers. These products help remove additional moisture from the hairs, making them easier to shave away.

- **Do you do anything to soothe your skin after shaving?** If the answer is that the client applies an **aftershave lotion**, your job is to tell him that although it may smell great, that burning sensation he feels isn't a sign of bravado but of skin stinging. The idea of an aftershave product should be to soothe and calm the skin, to feel refreshing but not burning. **(Fig. 8.5)** The best choices are **aftershave balms**, available in lotion, cream, or gel versions, and often with fragranced as well as unscented options. If a man's skin tends to be very dry, the worst thing he can do is use an aftershave; instead, he should use a gel-formula aftershave balm (look for the ingredients allantoin and aloe, which are especially soothing), bolstered by a moisturizer applied soon afterward.

- **Are ingrown hairs a problem?** You can probably answer this yourself by looking at the man's face, but asking allows you to let the man open the subject himself. A frequent cause is shaving over the same area twice, so alert the man to this factor. As an esthetician, it's your job to know how to remove ingrown hairs as delicately as possible.

INGROWN HAIRS: WHAT WORKS BEST IS WHAT'S GENTLEST

Many men try to remove ingrown hairs themselves and, in the process, make their skin condition much worse. In some cases, what was a **razor bump** becomes a full-blown infection. Ingrown hairs are basically hairs that grow back in on themselves, repenetrating the skin. Once it comes back into the skin, a hair is attacked by the body's natural defenses, just as any foreign body is, setting up the stage for later painful infection. Any man whose hair tends to curl may be especially prone to this problem. Ironically, the closer a man shaves, the more he may encourage ingrown hairs; only short hairs can reenter the skin once they have come out.

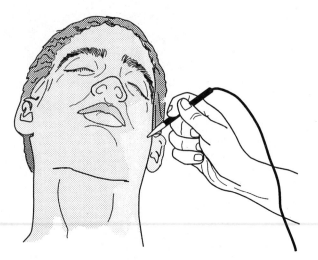

Fig. 8.6. Electrolysis can prevent severe ingrown hair conditions.

An esthetician can remove a few ingrown hairs with the help of a fine, sterilized needle and pair of sterilized tweezers. Gently try to flick out the hair with the needle, then to pull it out with the tweezers. If you don't succeed in two attempts, give up. Trying any further will only cause the removal of skin, which will leave a scar that may be more unsightly. Always follow with the application of a medicated drying lotion. Truly stubborn ingrown hairs should be cause for a referral to a dermatologist.

Recurrent, severe ingrown hairs may benefit from electrolysis. This is the conclusion of medical studies conducted by a dermatologist who was consulted by the Air Force to help them solve the problems of black servicemen (black men seem to be particularly prone to ingrown hairs, because of their hair's natural curl pattern) whose recurrent bouts of pseudofolliculitis prevented them from meeting the Air Force's clean-shaven requirements. (**Fig. 8.6**) This dermatologist found that electrolysis, using the more flexible **insulated bulbous (IB) probe**, could be successful in the destruction of ingrown hairs.

FASHIONS IN FACIAL HAIR: THEIR EFFECT ON MEN'S SKIN

The fashionable look in beards and mustaches—and whether to have them at all—varies along with every other fashion. Although it's not an esthetician's concern to set these fashions for individual clients, it is your job to help prevent unnecessary

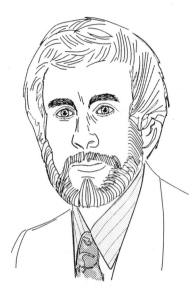

Fig. 8.7. Well-groomed facial hair.

skin problems. If a man has a beard or mustache, he must keep it as scrupulously clean as he does the hair on his head, to avoid skin breakouts or irritation from the natural oils produced by hair follicles. A beard or mustache can also easily trap foods or other dirt, so care must be taken by a man to wipe his mustache, for example, as well as his mouth after eating. This sounds simplistic, but an esthetician may be asked to explain skin flakiness or breakouts that are caused by less-than-ideal grooming of facial hair. (**Fig. 8.7**)

At the opposite extreme, the man who is obsessed with being as clean-shaven as possible may overdry his skin as a result. If a heavy five-o'clock shadow makes a man feel he must shave again before going out in the evening, suggest he use an electric shaver rather than a blade for that second shave, to lessen the chances of skin irritation. Many men find that giving their skin a "minivacation" from shaving on the weekends helps to heal red or irritated areas, making for smoother, easier shaves the rest of the week.

WHAT YOUR SALON CAN OFFER MALE CLIENTS

Along with advice on shaving, a skin care center can offer specialized services, such as **manicures** and **pedicures** for men, as well as gift certificates that the woman in his life can buy for him on special occasions. What else can you, as a salon professional, offer to attract and retain male clientele?

Keeping a Man Coming to a Skin Care Salon

COMFORTABLE HOURS Whether it's early morning or late afternoon sessions one day a week, flexible or extended hours are often a boon to busy executives, whether women or men. Don't overlook weekend hours, either—and not just on Saturdays. A few forward-thinking salons that are open on Sundays draw a surprisingly large male as well as female clientele for pre-brunch facials.

FATHER'S DAY FEATURES Special men-only packages—grouping together, say, a paraffin-mask facial and a pedicure—offered on days that will be for men only at a salon may lure those who would otherwise feel a bit squeamish, or tempt women to buy the men in their lives gift certificates.

MEN'S PRODUCTS A salon that claims to serve men as well as women but has skin care products geared only to women is doing its male clients a disservice. Make sure you can offer an appropriate selection to men, too.

ROUNDTABLE DISCUSSIONS Having an evening seminar on men's grooming may bring out those who are curious as well as those who are committed to taking care of their appearance. A skin care salon might co-sponsor such an event with a hairstylist, a men's clothing store, and an executive recruiter.

CLEARLY WRITTEN BROCHURES, FOR MEN AS WELL AS WOMEN You can't expect the women among your clients to suggest your treatments to a man if they don't even know such things are offered. Yet so many salons forget that the best place to promote the range of services offered is within the salon itself, by having lists of services posted in each treatment room and a variety of brochures available and easily visible in the waiting area and the front desk.

SELF-QUIZ: QUESTIONS TO CONSIDER

Is the daily ritual of shaving bad for a man's complexion?

Author's Advice: In fact, the act of shaving is a natural exfoliator, removing the uppermost, dead layers of skin and giving the skin a healthy glow. Of course, like any type of exfoliation, it can be taken to an undesirable extreme, which is the reason that properly preparing the skin for shaving is so important. Using the right cleansers as well as the proper shave preparation can help enormously to improve a man's complexion, and an esthetician can be the best guide to getting the best shave.

I live and work in an area in which men are still predominantly "macho." Will offering men's facials in a salon attract any clients around here?

Author's Advice: It might, but it probably should be approached slowly. Try having men-only evening hours or a men's day once a week. That way, the only other clients will be male, and men won't feel they are trespassing in a women's salon.

Also, be aware that the decor in the salon should probably be neutral in color and design. In certain areas of the country, men would be unlikely to feel at home in a salon with lots of flow-ery chintz sofas or pink walls. Don't forget the importance of all the accessories—towels, robes, etc.—not being in overly fem-inine colors either.

Many men in my area still believe that getting a tan is the best thing they can do for their complexion. How can I counter this?

Author's Advice: Try to make smart sun protection a part of any skin care con-versation you have with all clients, whether male or female. Don't overlook the importance of having samples of sunscreen products on hand in the salon; giving these to a new client to try can open up the whole conversation of sun protection without it sounding too forced or preachy.

Be careful, though. Too often, sun advice is ignored because it sounds like a cliché. Try to help each client choose the best sun protection products for his needs, geared to how much time he spends outdoors, what type of skin he has, and how much sun damage he has already. Stress the health dan-gers of the sun (the risk of skin cancer, especially) as much as the aging damage, so that using sunscreen is seen as an investment in health as well as appearance.

CHAPTER 9

The Anti-Aging Game:
What Skin Care Can Offer

It's no secret that we live in a society that is almost obsessed with youthfulness—and when it comes to a young-looking appearance, the skin is the number-one concern. Although it's true that the last two decades have seen a tremendous advance in knowledge about preventing and treating aging skin, it's also a fact that many claims are highly exaggerated. In this chapter, you will learn:

- what really causes skin to age
- how a skin care specialist can help clients preserve the look of youthfulness
- what a salon can and cannot do
- the powers—and potential dangers—of **deep-peeling treatments** and how to decide whether to offer them
- all-important advice to offer clients on caring for the skin at home
- what plastic surgery can do for your clients and how to help them, via skin care and makeup, to make the most of any surgery they decide to have done.

THE LOW-DOWN ON WRINKLES: GENETICS PLUS SUN

In the all-American zeal for self-improvement, cosmetics companies target anti-wrinkle creams at women in their twenties and beauty articles talk about the notion of "preventative face-lifts." In reality, the skin can begin to age ever so slightly as early as one's twenties, but such premature aging, science has revealed, is more often due to sun damage than genetics. Everyone will inevitably age, but those who have baked in the sun getting those glorious tans will inevitably age faster and more noticeably than those who sheltered themselves from the sun's burning rays. "When we're born, we get the skin that the good Lord gives us; when we're fifty and sixty and so on, we get the skin that we gave ourselves," comments Robert Auerbach, M.D., of NYU

Medical School. His all-important message is the one we all need to pass on to our clients: sun damage starts early, adds up over the years, and really starts to wreak havoc on the skin from age thirty onward. Using sunscreen—regularly and liberally—is the single best thing clients can do for their skin and their children's.

Just what is skin aging? The fine lines and deep wrinkles that we describe as old-looking skin result from the following changes:

- **Collagen**, the skin's texture builder, starts to degenerate. Skin becomes less plump.

- Elastic fibers become less resilient, thickening and literally decomposing. The skin becomes looser, sagging rather than hugging to the face and body.

- Oil—or **lipid**—production slows down over time. The good news is that older skin is less prone to acne breakouts than a younger complexion, but this decrease also means that skin doesn't retain water as well and becomes drier. Drier skin is not more wrinkly, but the lack of a smooth surface means that fine lines are more noticeable.

- Pores become dilated and more easily filled with debris.

- The ability to bounce back after skin damage, whether through bruising or overheating, slows down over time.

- After age thirty-five, the cell-replacement process in the skin's outer layer, the epidermis, slows down, with the surface cells remaining longer before being sloughed off. As a result, skin looks less smooth and even-toned.

Although everything previously described is part of a natural body process, studies repeatedly confirm that these age-related changes are accelerated by sun damage. Because it can take ten to twenty years for the cumulative impact of past sunburns and suntans to show up, the lines and wrinkles that appear and deepen in a person's thirties and forties may actually result from lack of sun protection at a much younger age.

Other lifestyle factors that can age a person beyond their years are **smoking, lack of exercise, stress, illness**, and frequent **"yo-yo" dieting** in which large amounts of weight are quickly lost and regained. Fair skin, which has less melanin, often shows signs of aging faster than darker olive or black complexions.

That doesn't mean that aging skin must simply be accepted. There are many treatments that can make tired skin look refreshed, revivified, and healthier. Scientific studies are confirming that it's never too late to start protecting the skin from the sun. Research at the University of Pennsylvania and other medical school dermatology departments has shown that sunscreen can not only protect the skin from future damage but literally give it a chance to repair itself from past damage. Combined with the expert treatments available in a skin care salon, that can result in rejuvenated skin for all of our clients. As with all skin care claims, though, it's important that we give our clients the most professional, expertly performed treatments. It is irresponsible to take advantage of fears of aging by making extravagant claims that a salon cannot fulfill. Also, because older skin can be more fragile, the expertly gentle "hands-on" style of each esthetician is especially important.

TARGETED FACIALS: MASKS AND AMPOULES

Certain simple steps can transform a traditional facial into a more skin-enriching treatment for older skin. None of these are meant to be pushed on clients, but they may be offered as part of a salon's services and suggested to those who ask if something can be done to help their skin more over time.

Light-Peeling Masks

Light-peeling masks can be used after the skin cleansing is completed to slough away dead surface cells, which are slower to "turn over" on their own after a person reaches age thirty-five. These are **enzyme-based** cream masks that can also be used by clients at home. The cream mask is applied to the skin, left on for ten minutes, and then washed off gently using warm-water-dampened cotton. These creamy masks are much preferable to the peel-off masks used by some salons because the cream, while being massaged off via the cotton, acts as a further skin slough. (**Fig. 9.1**) Peel-off masks, on the other hand, take very little of the skin debris off the surface and seem to be much ado with few results.

Natural Milk Masks

Milk contains protein, sugar, a whole range of vitamins, and pantothenic acid, all of which contribute to the renewal of skin cells, aid in preventing dehydration, and help strengthen capillaries. Some masks contain cheese or egg yolk, which are claimed to help prevent future wrinkles by bolstering the skin's natural protein. Milk masks are wonderful for nourishing skin that is becoming drier with age.

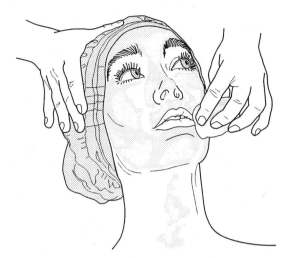

Fig. 9.1. Cream is massaged off with cotton, which acts as a further slough.

"Lifting" Masks

Acting as skin strengtheners, "lifting" masks contain ingredients that mimic the skin's own natural support chemistry. These treatments are recommended to be used twice a year, as boosters for the skin of the face and neck (a spot that's often ignored but where age lines can come early). Lifting masks are thus specially geared to those thirty and older, who are just beginning to see the impact of age on their complexions and want to encourage the skin to behave as younger skin does. The prime ingredients are **elastin** (the fibrous substance responsible for skin suppleness), **soluble collagen** (for deep hydration and line discouraging), and **hyaluronidase** (an enzyme that lowers the viscosity level of skin, allowing collagen and elastin to penetrate further).

Ionic Facial Toning "Lift"

This treatment is often described as a nonsurgical face-lift, since it so greatly minimizes the signs of aging, helping to "exercise" the muscles of the face and neck that help support young-looking skin. It utilizes a machine made by Bio-Therapeutic Computer Inc. that works on batteries; via cotton-tipped probes, the machine delivers a mild, pulsating current to the face and neck, helping to stimulate cell regeneration and muscle and tissue "firming." It's usually recommended for clients over the age of thirty, although some twenty-five year olds with severe sun damage could benefit from it, too.

Ampoules

Highly concentrated skin helpers packaged in small vacuum-sealed glass containers, ampoules maintain their freshness and potency until they come into contact with the skin. They can be used as part of a facial and also sold to clients for use at home. Two particularly effective ampoules are the **liposome mandarin booster** and the **kola nut extract ampoule**.

The **liposome** ampoule contains **organic mandarin extract**, **bee pollen extract**, and special **oriental mandarin extract**, combining the most modern technology of liposomes (literally little "bubbles" that carry active ingredients into the skin) with the purest botanical cosmetics. There are nine applications per ampoule, clearly marked on the container. A wonderful start to this treatment is to apply the first dose during a facial as the next-to-last step, under moisturizer, then to continue daily use of the ampoule under moisturizer. Skin should look fresher and smoother within three to six weeks.

The **kola nut extract ampoule** is rich in **amino acids** and trace minerals that help to brighten and revitalize a tired complexion. It is especially beneficial to skin that has become drier with age. Applied at night before bedtime to bare, clean skin, it should show visible results in two to three weeks.

THE GRADUAL PEEL: GLYCOLIC TREATMENTS

The rationale for offering anti-aging treatments often starts with one's clients. Those who routinely come for facials throughout the years often confide in salon personnel that they'd like to do something to help their skin a little more, to look a little younger and fresher. The after-effects of sun damage may be showing their first signs, with some fine wrinkling or leathery-textured patches. Your clients may even mention that they've been thinking about going to a dermatologist or plastic surgeon to see what could be done, whether they are good candidates for **Retin-A** or a **peel** or **dermabrasion**. The fact is that the majority of people who become steady clients of a skin care salon are interested in the latest advances for taking care of their skin. A responsible esthetician knows that when questions like these begin, it's the right time to tell a client about further services the salon can offer.

Glycolic treatments, which are gentle but effective skin restructurers, are a good first step for someone who wants to give the skin a visible boost. Through their gentle peeling action, they refresh the skin's outermost layer and go a long way toward waking up tired skin—at age thirty, forty, fifty, or beyond. They're also available in less concentrated at-home treatments, meant to be used alone or, for the greatest results by far, in tandem with salon formulas. Neither should ever be pushed on a client, but may be suggested to those seeking greater skin improvement beyond what a facial mask or ampoules can do. The client must understand that, because this is a light acid treatment, the skin will be a bit red for about three hours afterward. (Because of this, many people prefer to schedule their appointments at the end of the work day, so that they can go right home afterward.) The best results are achieved by repeating the treatment once a week for four to six weeks initially, with follow-ups once a month or every few months.

<u>NOTE</u>: Glycolic acid treatments should never be given to anyone without asking whether they are using Retin-A or any other topical or oral medication that makes the skin sensitive. It is imperative to ask every client about any prescription products he or she may be using beforehand. A person *can* combine the two but must use some of them less frequently while using the glycolic.

A salon treatment takes about fifty minutes; it is not a facial and should not be scheduled on the same day as one. The glycolic acid formula contains roughly 30 percent glycolic acid in a buffered base of chamomile and yeast; the pH of the liquid formula is 5.5. The face and neck are cleansed thoroughly, then massaged gently using a rich massage cream; (**Fig. 9.2**) the cream is then removed with wet cotton. There should be absolutely no steaming or squeezing of skin before the glycolic formula is applied. The client should be relaxed, with eyes closed and covered with cotton. You must inform the client that the formula will sting slightly when applied, but that this does not last. Three-quarters of a teaspoon of the glycolic formula should be applied with a cotton swab to the face and throat with extra special care taken not to get the solution anywhere near the eyes. (**Fig. 9.3**) The solution is left on the skin for ten

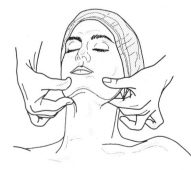

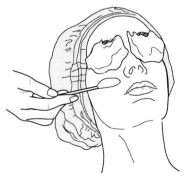

Fig. 9.2. Gently massage the face and neck using a rich cream.

Fig. 9.3. Apply formula to skin with a cotton swab.

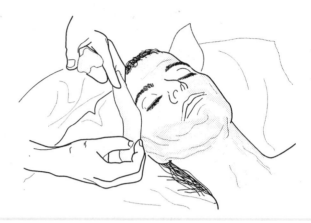

Fig. 9.4. Remove formula using cotton.

minutes and then removed very gently using cotton soaked in lukewarm—not hot—water. (**Fig. 9.4**) A lubricating, soothing oil containing botanical extracts called **Goldfish oil** is then applied to the skin with a spatula.   This formula, which comes in individual capsules, contains a soothing mixture of **ginseng extract**, **sunflower oil**, **apricot kernel extract**, **chamomile**, and **vitamin A**. The client is then left to relax for another ten minutes, to allow the nourishing botanical extracts to soak into the skin. A soothing moisturizer is then applied over the oil. Choose one that contains healing extracts such as aloe vera oil, hazelnut, yeast, and cornmeal.

As noted earlier, the client's skin will be a bit red for about three hours. No makeup or additional creams should be applied. To get the biggest benefit, the treatment should be repeated once a week for six weeks, then followed up with booster treatments every month or every few months.

The at-home version of the glycolic treatment is considerably milder, but also very effective. The results from combining the two options, at home and in the salon, can be especially grati-fying, giving the skin a super-fresh glow and smoothness. The at-home version comes in a cream formula that contains approx-imately 17 percent **glycolic acid** in a soothing base of **aloe vera gel**, **chamomile**, **witch hazel extract**, and **amino acids**. It is meant to be applied at night, after cleansing, twice a week for about six to eight weeks; once the skin is accustomed to it, it can be applied three times a week. This at-home glycolic cream can be an excellent alternative or supplement to Retin-A, since it is gentler and also helps smooth fine lines and resurface the skin to a new freshness, without the harshness or dangers of excessive sun sensitivity associated with Retin-A—and at a much lower cost to the client. Many clients begin using glycolic cream at age twenty-five or so. It can be as beneficial to oily skin as it is to dry, helping to soften the appearance of the first signs of aging, especially for those people who formerly were dedicated sun worshippers and are now starting to see the price show up on their complexions.

DEEP-PEELING MASKS: THE ULTIMATE SALON ANTI-AGING OPTION

For clients whose skin really needs a lift, who have uneven pigmentation, fine lines, acne scars, and/or sun damage, there is the option of a salon **deep peel**. These peels were developed in response to the peels and dermabrasions offered by medical professionals. The salon peel, done properly, is a much more gentle but highly effective treatment, dramatically improving skin tone, elasticity, texture, and coloration. Designed to remove the top four layers of skin over six consecutive days of treatment, the deep peel is the most intense form of facial treatment not offered by a medical doctor. Ideally, it should be done in the salon, but for those for whom this is impractical, it can also be done at home.

As previously noted in this chapter, the skin is constantly shedding and replacing itself, a process that slows down as we age. The deep-peeling treatment speeds up the process for dramatic improvement. Along with pepping up a dull complexion, it helps to remove impurities and tighten pores, giving the skin a new surface and younger and healthier looking texture. Because the results are dramatic, the treatment can benefit anyone—man or woman—over the age of sixteen who feels that their skin is in need of a significant boost. Benefits usually last about a year, although some deep-peel aficionados are known to show up at their skin specialist's door four times a year to give their skin a clean sweep at the start of each season. Done correctly, the treatment can literally be done every three months, as it does not pose the same severe challenge to the body's healing process that a more extreme medical peel does.

A typical salon peel formula contains **resorcinol**, **salicylic acid**, and **phenol** peeling agents, with the total concentration of these three ingredients at about 5 to 6 percent. The formula is buffered with vegetables, enzymes, and herbs. Some opportunistic suppliers might offer to sell more concentrated peel solutions to salon owners, but it is imperative that an esthetician not try to do a more severe peel—the risk that something could go wrong rises with the concentration of the peel solution. In fact, it is a good idea to be backed up by a dermatologist who is aware of the salon's peel formula and can provide advice or help if an individual client's skin seems to overreact.

It is important that you explain the following procedures, effects, and general information to the client before beginning the deep-peel process:

- The procedure involves application of the peeling formulation to the skin for six days, during each of which the client will spend roughly one-and-a-half to two hours at the salon.

- During the first three days of treatment, the client will feel a mild burning sensation for approximately five minutes after the preparation is applied.

- In the actual procedure, the skin is gently cleansed with cleansing lotion and warm water first; then the formula is applied using a spatula and the client is left to rest in a semi-darkened room. (**Fig. 9.5**) For the first three days, the esthetician should not leave the room until the preparation has been on the skin for about ten minutes and the burning feeling has stopped. The peel solution is then removed from the skin ninety minutes later by being gently sponged off with cotton and lukewarm water. (**Fig. 9.6**)

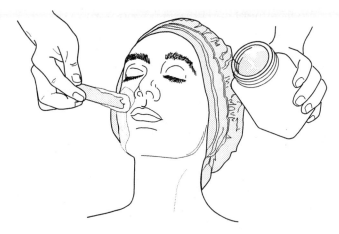

Fig. 9.5. Apply formula using a spatula.

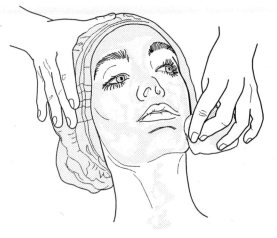

Fig. 9.6. Remove formula using cotton.

- There is no bleeding, scarring, or broken blood vessels, all of which are usual or possible in medical skin-resurfacing treatments.

- The clients must return to the salon for five more treatments. Their skin cannot be touched by *any* skin care or makeup products during this six-day regimen. This is an important point to emphasize before booking this type of treatment, because many clients will want to schedule it around taking time off from work (for example, having the first treatment Thursday evening and taking Friday and Monday off from work). The skin should just be splashed with warm or cool water and patted dry, gently, with a 100 percent cotton towel that has been laundered in a delicate, nondetergent cleanser. No moisturizer, no makeup, no soap, no shaving for the six days of the treatment.

- Clients should know that their skin will look as if they have been out in the sun during these six days. It will be slightly darker in pigment and on the fifth day will start to peel. It is vital that no effort be made to "help" the peeling process by rubbing the skin with a towel or washcloth, as that will only irritate it and delay healing. Sun exposure should be avoided for the duration of the treatment, of course, and for about six weeks afterward (it's a good idea to urge clients not to schedule deep peeling for summertime).

- Clients should be told not to exercise during the six-day period they are undergoing the peeling treatment, because sweat can irritate the treated skin.

- The skin needs extra-gentle care for the first week after deep peeling. A moisturizer containing **ginseng** and **collagen**, along with **vitamin E** cream, are recommended for use for at least a week after the deep peeling has ended. Clients should be urged to splash their faces with cool water as often as possible during this week. After that, regular cleansing and moisturizing, as well as makeup application, can be resumed.

- It is essential to ask clients, before scheduling this treatment, if they are taking any drugs that make them sensitive to heat or increase their skin sensitivity, or if they have any allergies to any of the ingredients contained in the formula. No one should combine salon deep peeling with the use of Retin-A or other medical peeling agents. It is standard policy to discourage anyone taking **antibiotic drugs** from having a peeling treatment, as the risk of blistering after even minimal exposure to **ultraviolet rays** is increased by antibiotics, and the peel treatment involves exposing new skin layers to the outside environment.

THE LIMITS OF SKIN CARE: WHAT SURGERY CAN OFFER

Although it is true that modern skin care treatments can do an incredible amount to improve the skin, it is equally important to recognize that making overly dramatic promises will only hurt your reputation in the long run. A deep-peeling treatment at the salon can lessen fine lines and stimulate new, fresher skin, for example, but it cannot tighten sagging jowls like a **face-lift** can. An intensive eye cream can help wake up a tired look, but it cannot get rid of undereye bags the way an **eye-lift** can. Similarly, a **chemical peel** at the dermatologist's office can penetrate much further into the dermis, more thoroughly resurfacing skin, than can a salon peel. Obviously, along with the benefits of medical skin treatments come certain risks not encountered in a skin care salon, such as the use of local or general **anesthesia**, the need for longer healing periods, and the use of certain anti-infection medications. A skin care salon should not view itself as being in competition with medical skin care and plastic surgery, but rather as being in cooperation with them. Thus clients can be helped to make the most of whatever treatments they desire by coupling a range of salon treatments with whatever medical anti-aging solutions they decide to try.

A working partnership, or referral situation, with one or more dermatologists and plastic surgeons in your area can improve the results everyone provides and can help to educate medical practitioners about the professionalism of skin care today. Because most medical schools offer no training at all about skin care, and many physicians still are male, the doctors literally have no practical experience in our field. A salon professional who becomes a resource to a doctor can help everyone achieve better results and can also gain a medical professional to go to should the salon staff members have any questions they need clarified.

Because so many clients of skin care salons do decide to pursue **cosmetic surgery**, it's important that the skin care professional have a basic understanding of what these procedures involve. An informed esthetician can help a client to make the most of cosmetic surgery by helping in pre- and post-operative skin care and makeup advice. Following is a quick guide to the most common cosmetic medical procedures, starting with peels and going on to body contouring.

Chemical Peel

When done by a dermatologist, a chemical peel usually involves **trichloracetic acid**; when by a plastic surgeon, **phenol** is more common. In any case, the peel strips away all the layers of the epidermis and the very top of the dermis. The result is equivalent to a second-degree burn, leaving behind very red, very oozy skin that literally stimulates the growth of brand new skin. The eventual results are quite dramatic, as surface lines, old acne scars, and liver spots literally disappear. Chemical peels are especially effective on sun-damaged complexions and are even sometimes used just around the upper lip.

A day or so after the peel is performed, a crust forms, which takes about a week to heal, after which it reveals much smoother, lighter, more sensitive skin. The new skin is very tender and it normally takes several weeks to return to its usual color. With a phenol peel, the neck cannot be treated, because the chemicals are so harsh that they tend to cause scarring in this area (phenol is also poisonous and so must be used with extreme care). The test of a good medical practitioner is that the treated skin is neatly "feathered" into the surrounding area, so there is no obvious line of demarcation. Darker skin tones, from Asian to Hispanic to Black, sometimes scar terribly, so some doctors refuse to perform peels on these skin types. Others have perfected techniques that can provide quite impressive results on deeper-toned complexions. Trichloracetic acid peels are sometimes diluted to the point where they are not much stronger than a salon peel; in this case, the results are also not as long-lasting.

Dermabrasion

Originally developed to remove acne scars, this mechanical skin sanding is now also used to treat wrinkled or sun-damaged skin. Dermatologists use tiny diamond-coated sanding machines to literally abrade away the upper layers of skin, totally removing all the layers of the epidermis to reveal the dermis, which then oozes and scabs and prods a new epidermis to regrow. Ten to fourteen days are usually needed before a person can be seen in public, during which time the crust gradually softens and falls off; painkillers are often necessary for the first day or two.

Dermabrasion is a traumatic experience for the skin. Consider the effect of a friction burn on your knee when you fall

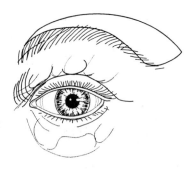

Fig. 9.7. The skin to be removed is marked.

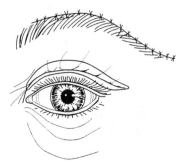

Fig. 9.8. The skin is excised.

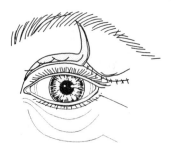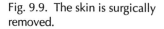

Fig. 9.9. The skin is surgically removed.

on the sidewalk—and then multiply that several times, all over the face. But results are also dramatic, as many people who have had the treatment can attest. In fact, it is one of the few options for truly improving deep, ice-pick-type acne scars. The skin is often red, tender, and easily irritated for several months. As with chemical peels, some doctors advise against this treatment for those with darker complexions, to avoid the risk of uneven pigmentation when the skin grows back.

Eye-Lift

This operation involves the removal of excess skin and/or fatty tissue either above or below the eyes; in some cases, both upper and lower eye-lifts are done. (**Figs. 9.7, 9.8, 9.9**) Although many cases are done on an outpatient basis, this is still major surgery. Bruising, swelling, and a black-eye look persist for a week or more, and it usually takes several weeks until the finished results can really be seen. Extreme care needs to be taken not to disturb the stitches at first, but that doesn't stop many people who have this operation from going back about their business surprisingly fast—especially now that wearing dark glasses in public, indoors as well as out, has become a fashion statement. The dark glasses, though, do more than hide the bruising from the public; the person's eyes are often very light-sensitive to begin with. **Camouflage makeup** can eventually mask some of the puffiness and discoloration as the person heals, but it's important to follow the surgeon's advice on when to start.

Face-Lift

Once a standard, simple procedure involving mere tightening of the skin, a face-lift can now be anything from simple skin

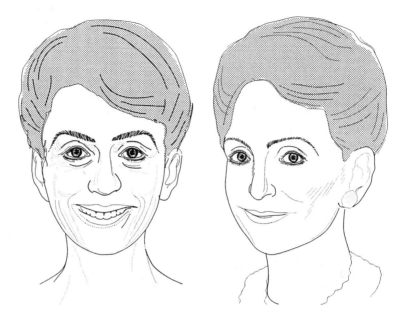

Fig. 9.10. Before a face-lift.   Fig. 9.11. After a face-lift.

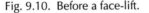

tightening to removal of fat, removal of excess skin, and literal tightening-up of the muscles that give the face shape and expression. Depending on the patient's age and degree of aging, surgeons customize this operation. Some doctors do face-lifts in their offices; others in hospital outpatient quarters; others in the hospital that require overnight stays. Stitches are usually hidden within the hairline as much as possible, but there is still a good deal of swelling, bruising, and discoloration during the first week at least. Care needs to be taken not to overdo anything, as much of the body's healing processes and circulation are directed to the face after the operation. (**Figs. 9.10, 9.11**)

Jaw-Lift

This operation, often done along with a face-lift when aging has produced a jowly effect, used to be limited to tightening up the skin. Since the advance of **suction lipectomy**, though, excess fat is also often removed, using a tiny, vacuum-like device inserted into the skin through a minute incision. The results really can be surprisingly dramatic—a firm jawline is an often-under-appreciated signal of youth. But while the firmness will eventually be there, the initial results are some swelling and puffiness that take time to go away.

SPOTLIGHT

Being in the skin care business for many years, I have come into contact with many well-known people, some of whom have been quite secretive about their lives and others who have shared an amazing amount of personal information with me. I had the opportunity to give facials to an actress who was incredibly vain about her appearance. In her midtwenties, she was already seeking out every anti-aging idea in the book. Although she was a regular monthly facial client at my salon, I knew for a fact that she also went to other salons and cosmetics counters seeking out anti-aging "cures." She used collagen creams, liposome facials, peeling creams, anything and everything that promised to make her skin look younger. Not yet thirty years old, she had the anti-aging mania of someone two to three times her age.

The year she turned twenty-nine, I didn't see her in my salon for four months. When she arrived for a facial, I immediately knew where she had been. Her skin was incredibly smooth and tight, and looked literally pulled onto her face—in fact, her usually radiant face had almost no expression! It turned out that she had finally found a surgeon who was willing to give her what she wanted: a chemical peel, collagen injections, and an eye-lift. Since I had not seen her in four months, I told her that I had to do a complete skin exam. Under the magnifying lens, I saw skin that looked incredibly fragile and sensitive.

I discovered I could no longer give her a facial massage without her skin reacting negatively. Just a few minutes of steam, on the coolest possible setting, and she started complaining that it was irritating her skin. From having healthy, vibrant skin that easily tolerated more creams and potions than most people could dream of, she suddenly had skin that was incredibly sensitive to everything. She soon discovered that she couldn't spend time outdoors because she sunburned so easily, even with SPF 15 or 20 sunscreens; chlorine irritated her, as did wind or heat. Over the course of the next few months, she discovered that almost everything she did seemed to irritate her skin.

She also began to question her own decision to search for an eternal fountain of youth. In seeking out perfect skin, she discovered, she had found skin that needed to be rigorously protected because it had been subjected to such severe treatments too early, before any damage had been done. Unfortunately, those who overemphasize anti-aging miracles often push people to do things too soon. Her experience made me realize that an overemphasis on fighting every sign of age could have a harmful effect on my clients. I hesitate now to suggest too much, but rather let clients come to me, asking for advice instead of being pushed to do too much too soon.

Filler Injections

Some of the most common anti-aging procedures are not technically surgery at all, but involve the injection of "filler" substances into fine lines and wrinkles. Some people have injections alone; others have both surgery and injections. The most common now are **collagen** injections. **Silicone** injections, although technically against the law, are still used by some physicians, although by fewer and fewer these days because its dangers have been so widely reported. Fat injections, using fat removed from the patient's own body, are also being used, as can mixtures of fibrous molecules combined with the patient's own blood components. All of these injections cause some initial puffiness that usually subsides within a day or two. They are often used around the mouth, above the lips, on the cheeks, or in the crow's-feet lines around the eyes. (**Fig. 9.12**)

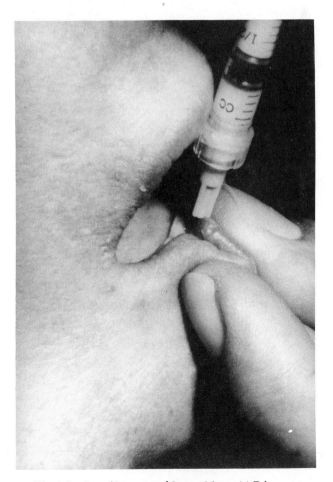

Fig. 9.12. A filler injection. (Courtesy of Steven Victor, M.D.)

HELPING SMOOTH THE WAY: WHEN A CLIENT HAS PLASTIC SURGERY

Although many people still prefer to keep cosmetic surgery a secret—saying, for example, that they are going out of town for a week or two—increasingly, estheticians are being confided in by patients who have decided to seek cosmetic surgery. This is all to the good, because a professional skin care expert can help a woman or man take the best possible care of the skin before the surgery and then gently nurse it back to health afterward. Surgeons routinely give out instruction sheets on caring for the skin before and after surgery, and an esthetician can help the client to decide which products are gentle enough to be used before and after surgery and which to avoid. You can also give instructions on extra-gentle cleansing techniques afterward. You will probably want to help a client to use makeup to mask some of the post-surgical swelling and bruising, as very few people can afford to stay totally out of the public eye for weeks after having surgery. Of course, you must emphasize to clients the importance of not applying any makeup until some of the healing process has taken place; for this, the client must follow the surgeon's post-operative advice.

Here is a quick guide to dealing with the after-effects of the most common anti-aging surgeries.

Post-Eye-Lift

Although eye-lift surgery eventually creates a larger area for eye makeup application, the lid will be swollen for many weeks, thus reducing the natural lid crease. To mask this, the makeup procedure should begin by applying an eye makeup base to the entire lid, which will help to conceal discoloration and keep makeup on longer. A very light-colored shadow should then be applied overall to further mask any lid darkness. A darker shadow should then be brushed on where the natural crease would be, to restore the natural shape of the eyelid that has been masked by the effects of surgery.

Under-eye swelling and bruising create a "black-eye" effect, which can be masked by using a concealer in a color one shade lighter than the actual skin tone. It should be applied with a sponge and patted on—never rubbed. To hold concealer on the skin, it should be dusted with a translucent powder afterwards. Avoid using very light shades, as this can produce a grey look; using too dark a shade will emphasize rather than minimize swelling.

Post-Jaw-Lift

The swelling from a jaw-lift will make the face look fatter initially, rather than streamlined. To minimize this until the swelling subsides, apply darker toned concealer to the jawline and chin to create the illusion of a more recessed area.

Post-Face-Lift

To mask bruising and swelling, use a concealer applied with a sponge under foundation and/or translucent powder. Use a damp sponge to blend the makeup so that there are no harsh lines of demarcation. Choose a translucent powder that has a bit, but not too much, shine, to counteract the dullness of swollen skin.

With all concealer applications, the makeup has to be maintained throughout the day. You don't want clients to overapply it in the morning, so the secret is to advise them to freshen it up at mid-day. It is a good idea to encourage a woman to carry a sponge and concealer with her in her purse.

Equally important to helping clients mask the initial bruising is to teach them new or slightly altered skin care and makeup techniques for after the surgery. This is an often overlooked reality. Makeup techniques, for example, that were used to "de-age" the face beforehand may be too heavy-handed for the post-surgery features. Eye-lift surgery creates a lot more space between the brows and the lash line, so new makeup techniques are especially essential. Skin that has been peeled is always slightly lighter in coloration, so there may be some need to adjust certain makeup colors, especially foundation. Salons that have a substantial clientele who seek out cosmetic surgery might want to offer specially priced post-surgery "makeup check-ups" that are shorter in length than standard makeup lessons and just focus on any adjustments to the client's makeup routine.

SELF-QUIZ: QUESTIONS TO CONSIDER

Many cosmetic companies sell peel-off masks that promise to slough off old skin, which clients ask about using at home. Are these a good idea?

Author's Advice: I don't believe in these because they don't do very much. They are a lot of effort for very little result. A better solution is to use a cream-based light peeling mask, first as a salon treatment and then as a follow-up twice a week at home. The cream is gentler on the skin but, because it can be massaged in as it is removed, it has the benefit of a more profound skin-sloughing effect.

Should all salons offer deep-peeling treatments?

Author's Advice: Not necessarily. These are specialized treatments that must be given with extreme care. The acids in the formula can be harsh on the skin if left on too long or applied too thickly, so an esthetician has to be committed to applying the peel solution carefully and following up on every stage of the treatment.

The majority of clients will want additional attention during a treatment such as this, so it's important not to oversell or over-book these treatments. A thorough medical history should be taken to avoid any contraindications, and clients need to be given a realistic view of what can be expected.

More and more clients, both men and women, are using Retin-A. Is this changing the type of skin care they need?

Author's Advice: Definitely. Skin treated with Retin-A is more sun-sensitive, heat-sensitive, and sensitive to all sorts of ingredients. It's important to take care to watch the skin for any reactions; if in doubt, be gentler than usual just to be on the safe side. It's also important not to use any bleach or waxing solutions on Retin-A-treated complexions. Be sure to emphasize how crucial it is to use a sunscreen to these clients, lest they unwittingly get bad sunburns.

CHAPTER 10 Makeup:
Supplying the Essentials

Although it is standard for just about every skin care salon to have a makeup area, there is nothing standardized about the way this area is set up and used. In some salons, it's a corner of a hallway where clients are offered the courtesy of do-it-yourself cosmetics; in large urban skin care centers, the makeup area may consist of several large, elaborately laid-out rooms that rival the sets of a top Hollywood studio. Makeup lessons may be a popular—and profitable—attraction. Whatever type of salon you own or work in, in this chapter you will find out:

- what a well-stocked makeup area should always include, regardless of size
- why cleanliness is so important, especially in makeup areas
- how the right lighting and seating arrangements can make a real difference to a salon's makeup success
- how to talk to clients about makeup.

SETTING UP THE SPACE

Even if a salon cannot devote a great deal of space to makeup, this is one spot in which utilizing space well is key. Nothing is less appealing than a slapdash approach to makeup display; everything needs to be neat and clean to a fault. That doesn't mean going to a great deal of expense; simple plastic containers that hold brushes, applicators, and small pots of makeup colors can be bought quite inexpensively. What is crucial is for the displays to be laid out neatly and freshened up after *every* makeup application. (**Fig. 10.1**)

One of the easiest ways to display various makeup colors and keep them organized is to mount them on plastic display sheets, either circular or rectangular in shape, with one tray for eye colors, another for cheek colors, another for all-over powders or cream foundations, and so on. A plastic lipstick case can be used to display all the lip colors available, and a plastic

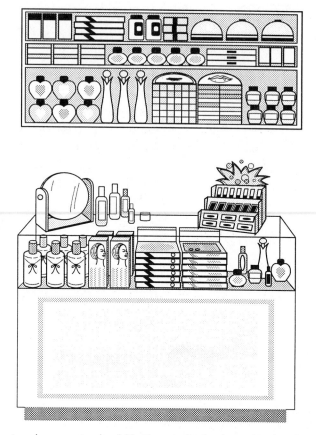

Fig. 10.1. A makeup center should be immaculately cleaned and well stocked after every use.

basket-type arrangement holds brushes and applicators (if you can't find one in a beauty supply house, consider using a picnic cutlery basket; it will work just fine). Foundations can be displayed on a tray or on a shelf (a good option if space is tight), but everything must be surface-cleaned after every single client. At least once every two months, *all* the products must be thrown out and replaced to ensure their freshness.

A nice-sized makeup room should measure at least five feet by five feet (of course, the more space the better); that way, two people—the makeup artist and the client—can be in the room without feeling that they are on top of each other. The mirror should be at least four feet wide so that the client can easily observe the makeup artist's technique from different angles. The stool for the client should be high and comfortable, preferably with a back that helps support the head (and hold it steady) for

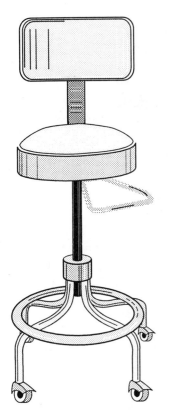

Fig. 10.2. A good makeup stool should have wheels and adjustable height.

application of eye and lip colors. Of course, the stool should be of adjustable height, as no two clients or estheticians are ever of the same size! The stool should also be on wheels, so that the client can be swiveled to different angles rather than having the makeup artist have to move around her. The most comfortable stools also have foot rests. (**Fig. 10.2**)

Although some makeup artists prefer to do their work standing up, a stool should also be available for the artist. She may want to sit down at some point, just for discussion, even if she still does most of her work while standing.

The lighting in the room is crucial to the end result of any makeup application. **Fluorescent lights** should be avoided if at all possible, because they tend to throw off skin and makeup colors. It's best to have natural lighting from windows wherever possible, or bulbs that are labeled "natural" or "high intensity" for the truest color. If bulbs are placed directly around the mirror, they should be on three sides only—never on the underside. Nothing stronger than forty-watt bulbs should be used (otherwise they give off too much heat). A **rheostat dimmer switch** is ideal for simulating different types of lighting—especially nice if you'll be doing someone's makeup for an evening wedding or other special occasion.

Finally, cabinets should be available for ample storage of supplies, so there's no need to run around the salon if something is used up during a lesson or application.

STOCKING THE SUPPLIES: WHAT'S ESSENTIAL

Having professional tools of the trade is what defines a makeup artist. In fact, some claim that the proper range of tools is more important than overly expensive makeup. You want to offer the best of both as much as possible.

As far as tools and makeup go, you want to have the following at minimum (**Fig. 10.3**):

- eyebrow tweezer (should be sterilized after every use and kept in a case)
- disposable sponges in round, square, and triangular shapes (to be thrown out after use)
- sterile cotton sheets or cotton balls
- cotton swabs
- facial tissues
- clips or headbands to hold clients' hair back (again, to be laundered or rinsed after every use)

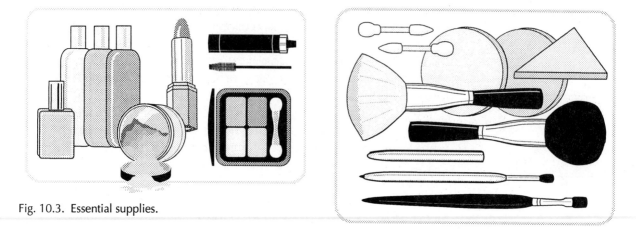

Fig. 10.3. Essential supplies.

Fig. 10.4. Have a selection of brushes and sponges available.

- cleanser, toner, and moisturizer
- foundation in as many shades as possible (a minimum of seven shades is essential; they can then be blended to match just about any skin tone). A liquid form is preferable if only one is available
- lipsticks (a minimum of sixteen colors)
- mascara (black, brown, and black/brown colors are all that's needed; other colors are strictly optional) and disposable mascara wands
- eye shadows (a minimum of twenty-five colors). If you have room for only one type, choose powder over cream or pencils
- under-eye cover sticks (three shades are usually the minimum)
- cheek colors (a minimum of six colors) in powder and/or cream form
- a selection of brushes for powder, eye shadow, cheek color, eye lining, and lip color (**Fig. 10.4**) (a minimum of six sizes).

Other options include a selection of eye pencils for lining and shadowing, lip-lining pencils in a variety of shades, gel rouges, foundation sticks, and eyebrow pencils. These are all extras that are necessary if makeup lessons are given, but not needed if courtesy post-facial makeup application is all that is done in the salon.

KEEPING EVERYTHING FRESH AND CLEAN

As with every part of the salon, cleanliness is a prime concern in the makeup area. This is especially true if the salon allows or encourages clients to apply makeup on their own after facial treatments; it is then essential to have a staffer check the makeup area after each and every client, because individual clients can make quite a mess of it, even in the most exclusive salons! Nothing will be as much of a turn-off to the next customer than to come out of a wonderful facial only to find a makeup-splattered countertop awaiting her.

After each client, any brushes that have been used must be replaced with fresh ones, with the used brushes taken away to be washed and air-dried. All disposable applicators should immediately be tossed in the trash can, and the countertop given a fast wipe-down to remove any stray makeup. Following are six important rules for keeping everything clean and safe:

1. **Use disposable mascara wands** *only*. Otherwise, you will have to sterilize the wand after every client. Even then, you run the risk of spreading infection if a staffer makes a mistake and fails to sterilize the wand after even a single client. The most dangerous tool in any woman's makeup bag is her mascara wand—she can even spread eye infections to herself. As any physician will tell you, sharing of mascara is a definite no-no, so wands should be disposable if at all possible, and each wand should get only one dip into the mascara container; if more color is needed to apply a second coat, use a new wand. **Conjunctivitis** (sometimes called "**pink eye**") is incredibly contagious, and a client can spread the infection before she even knows she has it. Recent research also reveals that some of the most dangerous diseases can be isolated from tears—reason enough to spend the small amount of extra money to use disposable wands. As professionals, it is our responsibility to protect ourselves and our clients.

2. **Lipstick should be applied with brushes** *only*. Again, certain surface infections can be unknowingly spread by allowing women to share lipsticks. In addition to using only brushes, saturate the brush with all the color you'll want so it doesn't need to be reapplied to the color—and use a clean tissue to wipe off the surface of the lipstick between clients.

3. **Use cotton swabs and disposable applicators for all eye makeup**. Again, this is wise to prevent possible spread of infections.

4. **Immediately replace any makeup that looks dirty, even if it's brand new**. This is for esthetics and safety.

5. **Every two months, replace all makeup**. Better to spend a little extra money than to end up with clients who develop rashes, infections, or allergies. Even with the most scrupulous attention to cleanliness, makeup is a natural habitat for bacteria. It's impossible to avoid something coming into contact with someone's skin, either the esthetician's or the client's, so along with between-client cleanups, it's essential to clean the makeup space thoroughly every evening and every morning, after the salon closes and before it opens.

6. **Discourage the use of fingers as applicators**. This is important to both makeup artists and clients. Wash your hands before and after each makeup application.

THE ART OF THE MAKEUP ARTIST

A big part of the makeup artist's role is in knowing how to talk to women about their appearance, to encourage them to use makeup to make the most of their features. This requires honesty, tact, and sensitivity. It is the esthetician's job to demonstrate what various products can do without false flattery or false promises. Makeup won't turn the typical woman into a model, but it can complement her best features. (**Fig. 10.5**)

Your role as a makeup artist begins with your own makeup, which should be attractive and professional. You should use makeup well, but don't overdo it. The idea is not to have every possible product on your face at once.

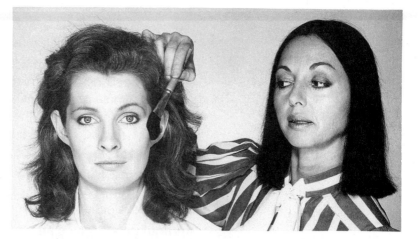

Fig. 10.5. Demonstrate your products.

SPOTLIGHT

Several years ago, I had one of the most rewarding experiences of my career by finding that makeup could help a woman's appearance better reflect her inner self. I had a client who had what could be called an "ugly duckling" syndrome. At the age of twenty-seven, she came to my salon for a facial, complaining that her skin "always had been awful, not like my sister's." Throughout her facial, she talked not about herself but about her sister—how beautiful she was, how pretty her clothes always were, how impeccable her sister's makeup was, and how easily she met new boyfriends. This client, whom I will call Terry, obviously had a poor image of herself and an oversized image of her sister.

In truth, Terry was a nice-looking woman, whose skin could use a little help and who could benefit from wearing a little makeup (she wore virtually none) and updating her clothes a little bit. I knew that I couldn't say this to her straight out, though; I had to wait for the right time.

After coming to my salon for several months for facials, Terry confided to me that she had trouble socializing. By this time, her skin was beginning to be in better shape and she obviously felt pleased with the results. I asked her if she would like to try to make the same improvement in her makeup that we were making in her skin. Little by little, I showed her different makeup techniques for bringing out her pretty facial features. First, I helped put emphasis on her eyes, which were quite gorgeous, by using a few soft colors. After she mastered the eye makeup techniques, I showed her cheek contouring and lipstick application. This not only made a difference in her appearance but, bit by bit, started to bring her out of her shell. Everyone in the salon noticed the difference in the way she walked in the door, no longer seeming to gingerly sidle in but walking in with a new look of confidence.

By the time she had mastered the makeup secrets, Terry was well on the way to equaling her sister. In fact, the next time she came for a facial, she told me about her most recent date, where she had gone, where the man worked, and so on. One day about a year later, she came into the salon and announced to me that she wanted to thank me for changing her life! She then told me that she was engaged to be married and that she felt she owed a big part of her happiness to the confidence I had helped her to discover. I was totally shocked but thrilled nonetheless. After she left, I thought back to the shy, plain-looking woman she had been two years before. That's what I like best about the skin care and beauty business, the chance to help people make changes for the best.

Whether a makeup application is done after a facial or as a separate service, the client's clothes should be covered to avoid getting them soiled and a band should be put around the client's hair to prevent getting foundation or powder beyond the hairline. The makeup artist should explain what she is doing as she applies products, with the goal not just of enhancing the client this once but of interesting her in makeup—which will bring her back to the salon either for additional lessons and applications or simply to purchase the products you have used and shown her how to use.

When makeup is applied after a facial, it is best to concentrate on the lips and eyes, explaining that the skin may be a bit sensitive and that the best treatment finishes up by allowing the skin to breathe free of too many products. All makeup applications should start with a discussion of the type of makeup the client usually wears, what shades and formulas, how much, and whether she wants a change. Ask if the client wants her eyebrows tweezed, and always tell her if the salon charges extra for this. The last thing you want is a client who says "yes," thinking the service is complimentary, if it isn't.

Always apply makeup to a clean face. If the application or lesson is not done after a facial, begin by using a creamy cleanser to wash the face; then use a toner, in the appropriate formula; and follow the toner with a lightweight moisturizer. Explain to the client that it's always best to use moisturizer under foundation to protect the skin and provide a base for the foundation to look smoother. If a woman says she never wears foundation (some don't), ask her why and see if you think it is appropriate. If she complains that it's because she can never get a color to match her skin, help her experiment with some. Be sure to apply the foundation test to her neck, both to get a better shade match and to check for any type of allergic reaction.

NOTE: Ask about any makeup allergies before embarking on a full-fledged application. If a woman is highly allergic, test products by applying them behind her ear and waiting a while.

As you apply makeup, keep the conversation centered on the client, explaining why you think specific shades or techniques will work for her. In the case of a lesson, the time should be split between your professional application of the makeup and the client's efforts. Many salons find that the best way to do this is to do only half of the face at a time. The client watches the makeup artist apply makeup to one side of the face, and then completes the other side herself, applying color to the second eye, the second cheek, the bottom lip, and so on. Be sure to emphasize blending of makeup throughout any lesson, since that is the single most common fault in most women's makeup application. One especially helpful feature of a lesson is to give the client a diagram to take home, showing where the makeup was placed and which colors were used. Many salons simply have photocopies of simple line drawings of a face on hand, on which the makeup artist can draw the colors she used. When available, small sample sizes of the makeup products used are also a nice giveaway at the end of a lesson.

SPECIAL PROMOTIONS: MAKING THE MOST OF MAKEUP

A modern makeup artist enhances a woman's best features and makes the artist's services pleasant, relaxing, and informative. There are also ways that makeup services can bring new clients to the salon or encourage clients to spend more time there. For example, many skin care clients in some salons don't even realize that makeup is available for purchase. A simple display of private-label products by the front desk is a discreet way of letting your clients know what's for sale. (**Fig. 10.6**) Although post-facial makeup application is usually offered as a complimentary service, clients who have a lot of questions should be politely encouraged to make a separate appointment for a lesson, during which all their questions can be answered in a calm, unhurried manner. Lessons can be offered

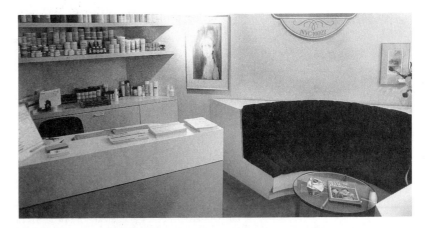

Fig. 10.6. Display private-label products by the reception desk.

in half-hour (one basic, everyday face) or one-hour sessions (the longer time can include a basic face plus evening special effects). Simple makeup application without a lesson can be priced lower. Some salons offer clients who buy a certain amount of makeup products (say $50 or more) one complimentary makeup application. Special-effects makeup applications may also be featured at an additional charge.

In the most innovative salons, special events are being staged in the makeup area. If there is room in the salon, special events can be arranged for holiday makeup applications or package deals featured for members of a wedding party. Children's parties (starting at four years old) or Halloween parties can also be featured. In short, the only limit is the makeup artist's and salon owner's imaginations.

SELF-QUIZ: QUESTIONS TO CONSIDER

Eyebrows are the frame of the face, so it's difficult to do one's best at applying makeup when the eyebrows are a mess and need a good cleaning and shaping. What can be done?

Author's Advice: You can politely tell the client that keeping her eyebrows groomed is one ingredient of getting her makeup to look the best—but don't push too hard. In most salons, eyebrow shaping is not a complimentary service, and you don't want to be perceived as doing a hard sell. You can, however, give the client a little bit of advice on the kind of shape that would work best for her face and eyes, and then ask if she would be interested in a professional tweezing, letting her know the cost. That way, you've offered information as well as a suggested additional service rather than just being a pushy salesperson.

How long should a good makeup lesson take? In the salon where I am employed, we're urged to make them as fast as possible.

Author's Advice: To give a woman a good idea of how to do her makeup herself, you need at least half an hour. A half-hour lesson allows the client to observe the professional's technique and also to give the application a try herself. Any less time and you really only have a makeup application by the professional, not a true lesson.

To try out special-effects techniques for evening or parties, a lesson should probably be about an hour long. Of course, the fee charged the client would also be higher in that case.

Rather than rushing to get makeup lessons over with as quickly as possible, at a low cost, a salon might consider raising its prices slightly and offering the clients more time. That way, the quality of the service would increase.

Are washable sponges a good idea for keeping supply costs down in a makeup room?

Author's Advice: Not at all. A wet sponge can easily become a breeding ground for bacteria, especially when it's used on more than one person's skin. Disposable sponges are really a must. To keep costs down, consider buying them in bulk if possible, as the price usually drops the more you purchase at once. And instead of buying various shapes, just buy only triangles, let's say, instead of round, triangular, and square sponges. This really isn't a place to cut corners by avoiding important sanitary measures.

CHAPTER 11   Being an Advisor:
*Teaching about
At-Home Skin Care*

One of the most important services you can give your clients is to help them take better care of their skin at home. After all, the time that a client spends in a salon is only a fraction of the time that is devoted to skin care in a typical person's life. Most of those hours are spent cleansing, caring for (or abusing!), or protecting one's skin on one's own. The better a client does on her own, the more you can do to keep her skin in tiptop shape—and the more she will appreciate the results that a skin care professional can deliver. In this chapter, you will learn how to:

- advise clients on cleansing, moisturizing, and protecting the skin
- give valuable advice and sell products *without* delivering a heavy sales pitch
- address special needs, ranging from sun care to teenage skin, aging skin, and skin care during pregnancy
- debunk the most common myths about skin care
- offer recipes for making low-cost skin care preparations at home.

BECOMING AN OBSERVER: HOW TO ANTICIPATE AND ANSWER QUESTIONS

Any smart businessperson knows that the first step to success is listening to the customer. Through questions and comments, your clients will let you know what they need and want. Listening to your clients also shows, first and foremost, that you care; even if you don't have all the answers, a bond is created through communication.

With each new customer, it is essential to find out what she or he does for the skin right now. Clients may tell you "nothing," but in reality that "nothing" is something. Do they wash their faces? With what? Do they use washcloths, towels, loofahs, cotton balls? Do they take off their makeup before exercise?

Before bedtime? Are they getting a lot of outdoor exposure? In winter? In summer? Do they work in an office or a factory? Do they spend a lot of time in overheated places? A florist's greenhouse? A chilly science lab? All of these questions provide essential information, and they are worth asking more than once. At least once at the start of each season, you should ask each client what she is doing right now to care for the skin, what type of makeup she is using, and what types of activities she is involved in.

The keys to at-home care are helping your clients to develop good skin habits, to eat well (not too much fat, not too much caffeine or spicy foods), to avoid smoking, and to avoid being too rough on the skin, either by picking at it or by using rough sponges or loofahs on the face. One strong point of salon services is the insurance they can provide that damage is noticed fast; it should be part of that service to find out what's causing the problem. Is air conditioning causing the surface of oily complexions to dry out and flake? Is a new exercise plan resulting in breakouts after years of clear skin? (In this case, a too-heavy moisturizer may be to blame for trapping perspiration against the skin.)

During the facial, it is each facialist's responsibility to explain every step—the masks, the moisturizers, and so on. This is also a perfect time to suggest some at-home steps that could help maintain each service's benefit, whether it be a weekly mask to use at home or a water-based foundation to help eliminate late-day shine. The majority of clients claim they don't want a skin care routine; they don't want to take the time or spend the money involved in using lots of products. But that's because the skin care industry has, unfortunately, created the impression through the years that the more products one uses, the better. Clients are often shocked when told that all that's involved in a preferred skin care routine is cleansing, moisturizing, and using sunscreen, but that's really the truth. Many clients want to try a salon's treatments for several months before investing in the products that are sold there. That's understandable, because they want to see results before they accept the whole program. Give them time and they will likely begin asking *you* for information about products, rather than your even having to suggest them. Salons that try to push too many purchases on their clients often lose rather than gain business.

CLEANSE, MOISTURIZE, PROTECT: THE MAGIC THREE

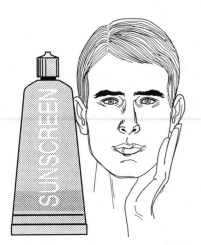

Fig. 11.1. Use sunscreen whenever outdoors.

One of the most common mistakes that skin care salons make is to develop a huge product line, matching all the commercial skin care lines, and then to urge a complicated mix of products on their clients. This is overwhelming, especially for a new client who may have done no more than use a bar of soap to wash her face in the shower each morning. That's why facialists should present skin care as three simple steps:

1. **Cleansing**. Whether you use a creamy cleanser plus toner, a bar-type cleanser, or a grainy scrub, the goal is the same: to get the skin as clean as possible.

2. **Moisturizing**. The choice of product here is key; it needs to be matched to your skin type and the demands of the climate or season.

3. **Protection**. For everyone, this means sunscreen whenever spending time outdoors. For some clients, it will also mean helping the skin to cope with the stresses of workplace environments, outdoor sports, indoor workouts, stress, or whatever. Protection can be a simple one-step solution or a more involved mixture of products to use depending on the time of year. The best advice is to keep this step, as well as the others, as streamlined as possible. (**Fig. 11.1**)

All of the additional products—masks, ampoules, intensive moisturizers, eye creams, night creams, body lotions—should be viewed as add-ons, to be introduced to the client when appropriate over time. They are not necessities for the skin care novice, and pushing them on clients too soon will only convince them of what they probably already believed: that skin care is too complicated anyway, so why try it? Instead, your goal should be to make smart skin care so simple that your clients will wish they had only found you sooner.

ADDRESSING SPECIAL NEEDS

There are specific times when clients need more than basic advice. For these clients, you need to be prepared to spend a little more time on explanation.

Pregnancy

Always ask female clients if they are pregnant. If they are, important precautions should be taken during the facial. No electrical equipment should be used, and less time should be devoted to steaming to avoid the woman's overheating. There should be more soothing—more massage, more cooling sprays—and be sure to put the woman's feet up.

It is also important to recognize if a woman is pregnant because of the changes that may occur in her skin. The elasticity may change slightly; pigment may deepen. (Some women literally develop the so-called mask of pregnancy, in which pigment pools around the cheeks and eyes. In such cases, you can offer advice on camouflaging makeup.) Sunscreen use is essential, as it can help prevent pigmentation changes in many cases. Seaweed masks are often a pleasurable alternative to traditional facial masks during pregnancy, as they are very calming to the skin, and can soothe any sensitivities.

The Sunny Seasons: Sunscreen Is Essential

Ask any client which is her favorite season of the year and she is more than likely to answer "spring" or "summer," the times of year when there's lots of sun and outdoor activities are possible. But those are also the times of year when the most damage can be done to one's complexion. In fact, the skin profession is always slowest in summer because people are afraid that a facial will fade their tans! (Nowadays, they may also be assuaging their guilt, knowing that the skin care professional will ask them why they got so much of a tan.) Customers are still incredibly naive about sun protection. They want to look better, which they think they do with a tan, but they don't want to look older, which is the inevitable result of sun worshipping over time. Some clients claim that they get as much of a tan early in the summer as they can in order to have more natural protection with the skin's darker color. Unfortunately, that's not the truth. (**Fig. 11.2**)

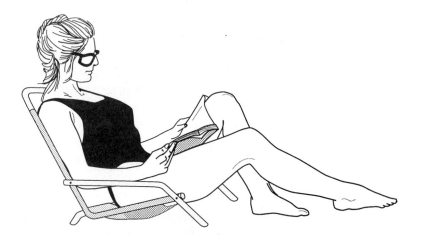

Fig. 11.2. Clients are still incredibly naive about sun protection.

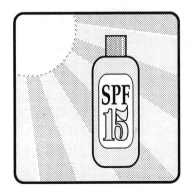

Fig. 11.3. Advise the use of sunscreen.

Until ten years ago, no one would listen to advice about sun protection. Just recently, more people have started using sunscreen on a daily basis. You should counsel your clients to use sunscreen instead of moisturizer as soon as spring starts—and to keep using it until fall is well underway. Even on cloudy days, the burning, aging rays are getting through. Many people use allergies to PABA (para-amino benzoic acid) as an excuse, but there are now many alternatives. **(Fig. 11.3)**

Whenever anyone gives you the opportunity to talk about skin care, you need to mention sunscreen. The sun is the biggest single danger to the skin, and no treatment, however wonderful, can really erase the damage. For those clients who do get too much sun, you can recommend simple old-fashioned remedies: a milk bath in which two quarts of milk are added to a bathful of warm water and the use of aloe-vera-gel-based skin soothers afterward (straight aloe gel from the health-food store is best initially, followed by a moisturizer rich in aloe). When clients come right after getting a sunburn, offer an in-salon treatment combining an aloe-and-seaweed mask for soothing with an oil-based moisturizing treatment (little or no steaming is used during this facial). Cool showers are advised, as is use of a milder (or no) astringent and continuous use of aloe-based moisturizers until the skin is fully healed. In cases of extreme sunburns, of course, advise consulting a dermatologist immediately. This is a must if there is any skin blistering, because prescription creams can help prevent post-burn infection or scarring.

SKIN MYTHS: THE SUPER SIX

There are certain misconceptions about skin that seem to endure, year in and year out, cutting across generations and different cities and states. Gathered here are the top six questions that estheticians seem to hear the most frequently.

1. **Do I really need to take my makeup off before I go to sleep?** Believe it or not, there are women who still don't understand that the skin needs a rest from makeup, just as their bodies need a rest from activity, and that the dirt that accumulates from a full day's activity needs to get washed away as well.

2. **Should eye cream be applied to the top lids as well as the bottom?** For some reason, many people recognize that the under-eye area needs special care but don't acknowl-

edge that the eyelids also need special attention. Don't just push the sale of eye cream or gel; tell your clients how and when it is to be applied. Otherwise, you're doing them a disservice.

3. **Should I always apply moisturizer under my makeup?** Although foundation formulas have gotten more "skin-friendly" through the years, most skin care professionals still agree that a thin layer of moisturizer should be applied to the skin first to act as a buffer between bare skin and makeup. This is especially important if skin is sensitive or dry, because even a creamy foundation formula doesn't contain enough moisturizing ingredients.

4. **Do I really need to apply moisturizer to my skin before steaming it at home?** All too many home-steam aficionados risk micro-injuries to their skin through overzealous and careless use of home steam machines. The tell-tale signs are broken capillaries, reddened skin patches, and sunburn-like areas at all times of year. It's hard to break old habits, but this is one you should try your best to discourage. If a person really likes to steam her face at home, she must be as or more careful than we are at our salons—and professionals *never* use a steam treatment on bare skin.

5. **Why do I need to take my makeup off before exercising? I thought sweating naturally cleaned the skin**. This is a true cleaning only if the dirt and toxins are allowed to escape through the pores—and pores covered with makeup don't allow much escape. When skin looks very sensitive or irritated, this is often a secret culprit.

6. **Is swimming really bad for my skin?** Chlorine is a well-known damager of hair, but few people recognize that it can also dry out the skin. That's why I urge swimmers to lavish on moisturizer and/or moisture-rich sunscreen formulas (if they do their swimming outdoors) and to rinse off as soon as possible after swimming. It's true that exercise is great for the complexion, boosting circulation and moisture supply, but chlorine isn't.

AT-HOME SKIN CARING: A COOK'S CABINET

One of the most common questions asked of estheticians is whether natural or homemade skin care products are better for

SPOTLIGHT
••••••••••••••••••

When I grew up on a kibbutz in Israel, there were sources of natural nourishment, for body and skin, all around. At around the age of fifteen or sixteen, my friends and I would use our spare time, in the evening or weekends, to concoct our own skin preparations. The reasons for this hobby were several: a desire to beautify ourselves, combined with a lack of money to buy expensive cosmetic products and the availability of a range of natural ingredients right outside our front doors.

Among the preparations we cooked up were banana and avocado masks, sour cream and strawberry masks, pineapple compresses for our eyes, and cucumber and grape cleansers. We didn't have, or know about, sunscreens, so we often used soothing milk-based cleansers to try to erase the freckles we would inevitably get from spending our days in the sun. We drank a lot of water, because it was hot and fresh, cool water was always available.

When I entered the skin care business years later, those home lessons served me well. The more I learned about the science of skin care, the more research began to turn up about the powers of natural ingredients for at-home skin care. I would love to be able to prepare custom-made natural products for each individual client, but of course that isn't practical. Freshly made cleansers and masks have a very short shelf life and take too much time to be able to mix for each customer. In an effort to continue that tradition, though, many of the products I have made for use and sale in the salon contain these same natural ingredients, as do the products of many other cosmetic companies. To make them more practical, they also contain certain other ingredients that help them last for weeks rather than days.

I haven't given up on my natural-cosmetics background entirely, however. I still offer my clients recipes for making their own products at home and find that it is still something I myself enjoy doing when I have the time—although with running a business and being a mother it isn't as often as I'd like. But even after all my years in the business, I find that there is an added element of relaxation to taking care of one's skin at home with ingredients that have been mixed up in one's own kitchen. It's a pleasure I encourage every skin care professional to share with her clients.

the skin than the store-bought variety. Although the most important factor is to use products that are appropriate for an individual's skin type, many homemade skin cleansers and tonics do add to the pleasure of taking care of one's own skin and can also help the results. They may not be better, but they are a pleasant alternative. (**Fig. 11.4**)

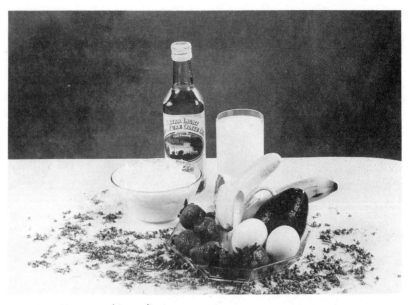

Fig. 11.4. Use natural ingredients.

CAUTION:

- Review the recipes carefully before mixing ingredients.
- Label all storage containers.
- Store all recipes in the refrigerator; discard after two weeks.
- Never leave products at room temperature for longer than it takes to use them.
- Perform a patch test prior to applying complete mask. Discontinue use of product should any reactions occur.

Facial Favorites

The following two cleansers are meant for the face only:

Cucumber Milk Cleanser (for dry skin)
Use a blender to liquify one cucumber; strain to remove seeds. Mix together equal amounts of cucumber juice and whole milk. Apply to skin with cotton ball and rinse immediately with cool water several times. (Can be stored in refrigerator and used over the course of *one* week only.)

Almond Milk Cleansing Lotion (for oily skin)
Put 1/4 cup almonds into food processor and process into almond meal. Blend together almond meal, 3/4 cup **rosewater** (available in health food stores or

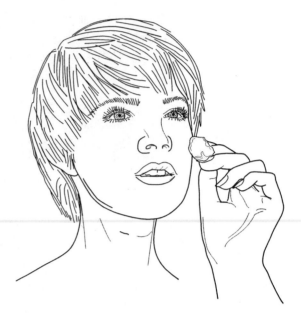

Fig. 11.5. Apply to skin with a cotton ball.

beauty emporiums), and 1 tablespoon witch hazel. Apply to skin with cotton ball and rinse immediately with cool water several times. **(Fig. 11.5)**

Most Effective Moisturizer

As with store-bought moisturizers, this should be applied to clean, bare skin with the fingertips. It is intended for the face and can be worn under makeup or alone, or used as a refreshing lightweight night cream.

Sensitive-Skin Moisturizer (also can be used by new mothers)
Warm 3 teaspoons honey in a double boiler. Remove from the heat and slowly add 1/2 cup almond oil and 1/2 cup avocado oil (available in health food stores or supermarkets). Drop by drop, stir in 3 teaspoons rosewater. (Keep refrigerated for one day before use; discard after two weeks.)

Skin Toners

These should be applied to skin after cleansing.

Dill Astringent Lotion (for all skin types)
Boil 1 cup fresh dill in 2 cups spring water. Allow to cool; filter through a fine piece of cheesecloth. Apply to skin with soft cotton ball. Can be rinsed off or left on the skin.

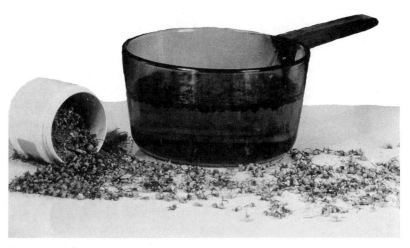

Fig. 11.6. At-home recipes.

Blueberry Tonic (for normal-to-oily skin)
Mix together 3 tablespoons stemmed, crushed blueberries and 1/2 cup sour cream or plain yogurt. Apply to face and neck and rinse off after a few minutes with tepid water.

Natural Melange Masks

Giving oneself a mask at home is always a chance to put one's feet up and relax. Here are two all-time favorites.

Grape Mask (for dry skin)
In a blender, blend 1 cup seedless grapes (red or green) until pulpy. Apply to face and neck before showering; leave on about five minutes. Rinse off in shower with warm-water splashes. (This is a perfect once-a-week skin reviver.)

Avocado Mask (for all skin types)
Mash 2 tablespoons avocado; blend with 1 tablespoon honey and 2 drops lemon juice. Apply to clean skin; leave on for 10 minutes. Rinse off with lukewarm water. (**Fig. 11.6**)

SELF-QUIZ: QUESTIONS TO CONSIDER

A new client arrives for a facial and you casually ask, "Please tell me how you take care of your skin." Her answer is, "Oh, I don't do anything." And then she refuses to say anything else. How would you broach the subject of what to do at home with this client—whose skin is obviously a bit dry and irritated, probably the result of using too harsh a cleanser and/or not moisturizing enough?

Author's Advice: The best way to approach any subject with someone who doesn't seem eager to discuss it is gently. The best opening lines are usually gentle praise, which will put the client at ease and show her that you don't intend to barrage her with a sales speech. I would start by saying something like, "You know, your skin really looks beautiful, you don't have any breakouts or rashes, but we all need to be aware of the way that the environment is affecting us. I've found that moisturizing more can really help keep the skin smooth and fresh."

The idea is to make a conversation out of it, not a lecture. You've raised several topics—the environment, moisturizer, rashes—all of which may prod the client to respond in some way, which then keeps the dialogue open and gives you a chance to gently mention what you think would be best for her skin. But don't force the subject. If a client truly does not want to discuss at-home care, just concentrate on giving the best facial you can. Eventually, she will probably ask you about taking care of her skin at home, and by that time you will have proven your expertise in her eyes.

In many salons, the facialist gives each client a list of products suggested for home use. Is this a good idea?

Author's Advice: I think it is, and often use this technique. The facialist must be sure to explain that these are some suggestions appropriate for the client's skin type, and that the client is welcome to discuss the list further with the manager or salon owner. All products should be listed with their prices, so there are no surprises. If the customer says that she doesn't want all this fuss, the manager or owner can suggest the two most important products that will provide the greatest benefits with the least amount of fussing.

It is also crucial that the facialist, manager, and owner all make it clear to the client that any questions that come up during at-home skin care can be answered by simply phoning the salon. No products should be sold without this type of customer support.

Many clients in my big-city salon complain about how dry their skin becomes because of overheated apartments and air-conditioned summer homes and offices. What is the solution?

Author's Advice: A noted dermatologist once said, "The same environment that is ideal for houseplants is ideal for the skin." His point is that skin smoothness benefits from a greenhouse environment, which means surrounded by warm, moist air. In fall and winter, when steam heating of houses and offices robs the air of moisture, I suggest to all my clients that they use a humidifier to boost the moisture content of the air. In fact, for people who complain a humidifier doesn't make much of a difference, I even suggest an old-fashioned vaporizer, which emits a warm mist. Often, just several nights of sleeping in a room with a vaporizer makes a difference in skin's texture.

PART II
SKIN CARE BUSINESS SPECIFICS

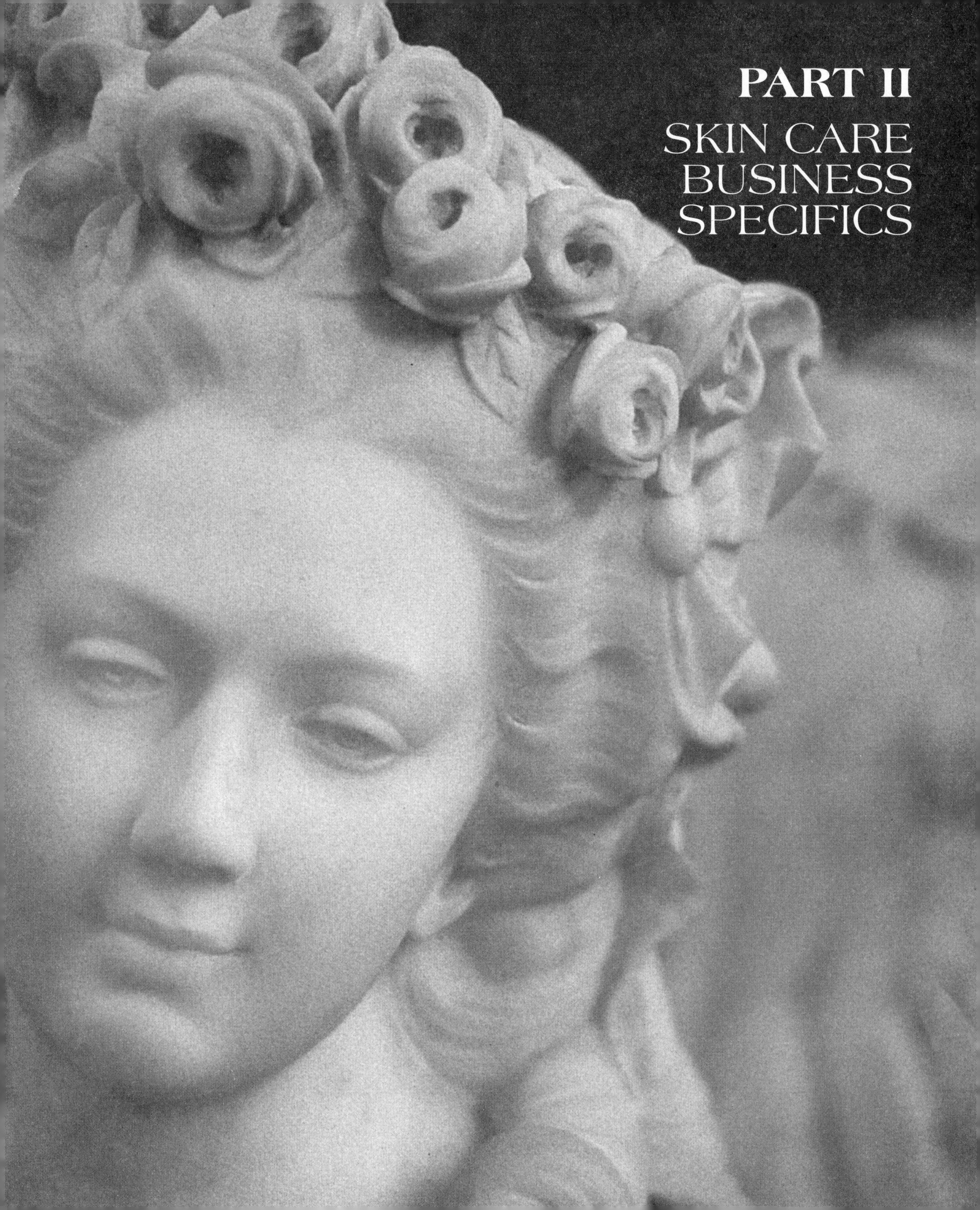

CHAPTER 12   The Esthetician's Image

The elements of an esthetician's job involve everything from providing personal service to presenting an image for others to aspire to, from sharing and giving to others—in terms of information and self-esteem—to operating a business. In a business geared to helping other people make the best of their appearance, it is absolutely incumbent upon all of us to look as good as we possibly can. In this chapter, you will learn:

- to understand the importance of personal hygiene
- to balance your own sense of personal style with the style of the community in which you work
- how to find the job possibilities open to trained estheticians
- how to prepare for job interviews and work your way up within the field.

HYGIENE: THE VITAL STARTING POINT

A professional esthetician should be a personal example of good health and personal grooming. The most crucial image concern for any esthetician isn't the color of her eye shadow or her lipstick but her own personal grooming. Good oral hygiene, cleanliness, good posture, a balanced diet, and good sleeping habits are more important than the latest fashions. Image doesn't stop with the surface: intelligence, integrity, compassion, and enjoyment of one's career all contribute to the image that each of us presents to our clients every day. In fact, personality is a good part of any esthetician's success. A person who enjoys the job and greets her clients with a positive attitude is more likely to develop a loyal following than is the best technician who has little personality.

Hygiene, though, can destroy the most promising of careers. The reality in our jobs is that we are under stress and often work in warmly heated environments, and thus do sweat. Add to that the fact that we wear mostly nylon uniforms over our clothes, and you can see that deodorant is a must. You can't just change your uniform a few times a week and expect it to smell fresh and clean. Daily change of uniform is essential. At the start of one's career, even someone who purchases just one uniform can rinse it out in a basin of cold water and gentle cleaner at night and hang it up to dry by the next morning. Breath spray, soft makeup, and hair that is brushed or pulled back off the face are also important.

Remember that an esthetician is responsible to the public in the salon. If you have a bad cold or cough, don't go to work that day. You will only spread your germs throughout the salon and alienate people who don't appreciate paying to have someone sneezing or coughing in their faces. For minor sniffles, be sure to have plenty of tissues on hand in each treatment room (they come in handy, too, if a client has a cold). Try to get enough sleep; feeling and looking tired doesn't inspire confidence in one's abilities. Brush your teeth twice a day at a minimum. Wash hands before and after *every* client. Avoid the sharing of towels in the salon by using paper towels; the hands are one of the most common routes for spreading of cold and flu germs.

DRESSING ON THE JOB

The beauty business is a fashion business, but that doesn't mean that an esthetician has to be a slave to fashion or spend every cent of her hard-earned money on constantly buying clothes. What you should aspire to is a clean, well-groomed look that reflects an awareness of fashion but not faddery. You need to be aware of the fashion trends in your area; what passes for the height of chic in New York City might seem ridiculous in Phoenix, and vice versa. Pay attention to details. Be sure that your shoes are well cared for; if they need heel lifts or polishing, be sure it's done. Always carry an extra pair of pantyhose in your purse so that if you do get a run you can change into a fresh pair. If you like wearing jewelry, you can wear it, but beware of anything that gets in the way of delivering the best possible service. You don't want overly jangly bracelets that make so much noise the relaxing facial massage you were giving turns into a noisy percussion band. The same goes for overly large, overly noisy earrings that jingle with your every move. Most people prefer to keep the rings they wear to a minimum when they're working with creams and lotions. Choose colors that flatter your own coloring; they can be bright and cheerful if you wish, but not overly loud.

MAKING BEAUTY A PROFESSION

One of the questions most commonly asked by those considering becoming estheticians is whether there are really job opportunities out there. The answer is yes, now more than ever. Unlike other professions in this country, the beauty business has truly grown, as part of Americans' continuing interest in health and fitness from the inside and out. There are virtually unlimited opportunities for those pursuing an esthetician's license nowadays. Americans have become more aware of skin care, sales of grooming products are now a multimillion-dollar business, and cities that had only one skin care salon during the 1970s now have tons listed in the phone books. In 1969, there were a handful of skin care salons in New York City; as of 1993, there were at least fifty salons exclusively devoted to skin care, and probably half of the hair salons now offer other beauty services as well. All across the country, hair salons are offering esthetician's services, in some cases even expanding their facilities to make room for beauty services.

All of these places need experienced estheticians to offer beauty services, and they're not alone. An esthetician can choose to specialize in corrective therapeutic makeup, working with physicians who treat victims of burns or congenital deformities. One might specialize in pedicures and manicures, even opening a salon devoted solely to hands and nail care. Another esthetician could be a salesperson for a beauty supply company or top-of-the-line cosmetics company, selling the product to department and specialty stores. You can switch jobs within the same career, becoming a cosmetics buyer for a department store, for example, or working at trade shows in which companies show their wares to the beauty field. One can do image counseling, color consulting, work for or become a makeup artist, a receptionist in a salon, a salon manager, or pursue further education to become a cosmetic chemist, working for a major cosmetics firm or a private-label cosmetics house that produces products used in skin care salons across the country and around the world. Manufacturer's representatives who call on salons, drugstores, and department stores need to know about the products they are selling; someone with an esthetician's degree can do much better sales presentations than someone who has little or no knowledge of what they are selling.

Esthetics can be combined with a nursing degree to work counseling patients in hospitals on the importance of appearance;

for example, the American Cancer Society now has a "Look Good, Feel Better" program in which estheticians work with recovering cancer patients to help them appreciate the difference that looking better can make to eventually feeling better as well. Dermatologists and plastic surgeons often rely on the nurses in their offices to offer beauty advice, but are now increasingly turning to estheticians in private practice. Combining the two areas will be a lucrative move in the future, as more and more people age and seek out cosmetic surgery to look as young as they feel.

In short, the possibilities are almost endless, but it's important to remember that professional training is a must.

Have Diploma, Will Travel

In the United States, it is still common for hairdressing and esthetician's programs to be combined into one in schools. A hairdresser has to be licensed as a cosmetologist in most states first. In most states, esthetics is not a separate license, but it is a separate diploma, received by doing additional study after one receives a cosmetologist's license. A hairdresser can specialize in color, scalp treatments, and haircutting for women or men; a facialist needs a skin care diploma that indicates further specialized study. Makeup artists do not have to be licensed in this country, but a makeup artist should have an esthetics education to do the job properly.

Getting an education is an important first step and is also another possibility for those who are seeking to switch careers. Who better to become a teacher at a technical school than someone who has had a long career in the field? In fact, considering teaching is a great way to refresh one's interest in a field, because the challenges of explaining information to young people is often the best possible refresher course.

Job Interviews: Being Prepared Is Key

Always prepare for a job interview by doing your homework. Find out as much as possible about the company you are applying to ahead of time. If the company is big enough to be written up in magazines or newspapers, go to the library to do some research. If you know anyone else who has worked there, make some phone calls and ask questions.

Call a day ahead to confirm your appointment. The day before, prepare all your diplomas and certificates to bring with you. Bring any letters of recommendation with you or bring addresses and phone numbers of those who are willing to provide you with references. Bring the addresses and phone numbers, as well, of any schools you attended. To show that you are truly ready to start, bring your uniform and tools (personal tweezers, makeup brushes, whatever) in a little bag; you never know when some overbooked employer will say, "Let's give you a try." Arrive a little before the scheduled time so that you can wait, but don't keep the potential employer waiting.

During the interview, listen to what is being said to you before you volunteer endless information about yourself. If you don't understand something, ask for a fuller explanation. Act enthusiastic and, when asked questions, do sell yourself. Remember that this is your chance to present yourself and to shine. Don't be shy; try to project your best qualities. Present your knowledge without lecturing, and keep all your comments upbeat and enthusiastic. Ask questions that show you've thought about the kind of job you would like and the kind of place you would like to work. Be honest; if you lack experience in a given area, admit it, but turn it around by adding, "But I'm a fast and enthusiastic learner." Don't be shy about your willingness to learn whatever is required for a job you would really like to have.

HUMAN RELATIONS: THE PSYCHOLOGICAL ADVANTAGE

Anyone who is experienced in skin care knows that it is probably one part technique matched by one part attitude. The way you make your clients feel about you (and themselves) is as important as any treatment you give their skin. A good esthetician needs to project a positive attitude, to be gracious and polite with clients, to be friendly and interested in them without being nosy, and to make them feel at home in the salon. Clients will trust you more with skin care advice if you act sincere, show your intelligence, and greet clients as if you were welcoming them to the salon for the first time every time. Don't act as if you take their coming for granted because before long, they won't be coming anymore. A skin care salon is a place where every client should feel truly special.

It's inevitable that skin care salon personnel learn a lot about their clients; often, we are the recipients of confidences from our clients. It's vital to maintain a professional attitude, though. Don't pry for more information; just listen to what's volunteered and react with empathy, but don't try to give advice that you're not qualified to offer. When striking up conversations, try to avoid politics and religion; the last thing you want to do is get into a passionate argument with a client. Don't bring up your

SPOTLIGHT
••••••••••••••••

When I arrived in the United States soon after completing my cosmetology degree in Israel, I discovered that I would have to become licensed as a hairdresser to practice my profession in New York state. I went to school and managed, with my fractured English and all, to pass the exam at the same time that I was completing thorough training in English language courses. Since I had gotten a taste of hairdressing, I decided to give it a try, and applied for and got a job in a small hair salon in New York City. After two months on the job, during which I did everything from shampooing clients' hair to trying my hand at haircoloring and cutting, the owner asked if I would like to make a move up, to managing a smaller salon he also owned in another neighborhood. This salon, he explained, had a steady clientele and was a good training ground for someone who was interested in being a businessperson.

I agreed, nervously, to give it a try. To my surprise, I enjoyed the chance to run my own show. When I didn't know the answer to a question, I simply called my boss at the other salon to confer with him. But what I didn't like at all were the fumes that were inevitable at that time in a hair salon; the chemicals from the heavy perms, hair dyes, and frostings made me sneeze and my eyes water constantly. I realized then that the hair salon business wasn't for me. Also, I really missed skin care, my true love as a profession.

This was the 1970s, when the number of skin care salons in New York City could be counted on less than the fingers of one hand. Through persistence, though, I managed to get an interview with one of the biggest names in town. I was incredibly nervous the night before, going over and over what I should wear (I changed my mind at least a dozen times and almost went out to buy new shoes and a dress that very morning!) and how I should style my hair and what I should say. The woman who interviewed me lived up to every expectation and more: she was gracious, intelligent, beautiful, and warm. She smiled a lot and tried her best to put me at ease—I am sure she could see my knees shaking. She asked me questions about myself and gave me a chance to talk about my hopes for the future within the skin care profession.

At the close of a lengthy conversation, however, she told me that she had truly enjoyed meeting me, but that she had no openings at present, and that I really needed to get some experience in the skin care field in the United States. To this I replied, literally without thinking, "You don't even have to pay me, but please let me work for you." The honesty of my remark must have caught her off guard; she announced that she could offer me a part-time position of a few nights a week from 5 to 9 P.M. I said yes gladly, even though it meant a one-and-a-half-hour commute each way to and from Brooklyn.

After four months of part-time work, I got a phone call at home one morning. My boss informed me that she now had a full-time opening, and that because I had shown such dedication to my part-time position, she would like to offer it first to me before anyone else. I accepted with joy—and went on to make skin care my profession and to model my own career after the "big names" of skin care, eventually opening my own salon.

This experience taught me that, in going after something you want in your career, honesty is truly the best policy. I knew that I truly wanted experience in this profession and literally would work for nothing (although happily I did not have to) in the hopes of getting it. It was also proof that showing one's interest and enthusiasm is the best way to qualify for any job opportunity. People who have dedicated themselves to a field look for that type of dedication in others.

own problems, even if they're similar (or worse than) the clients'. And in no case complain about other staffers or make sarcastic remarks about other salon clients. *Never* spread gossip; it will only backfire on you in the long run.

Courtesy and Respect: What Every Client Deserves

Treat every client like a VIP. Project that idea with courtesy and patience. Be helpful to everyone. In business, try to remember the idea that the customer is always right; even if one is not, try to solve the problem with as little annoyance or inconvenience to the client as possible. If in doubt about how to handle a situation, call on the manager of the salon, in a friendly manner, for help. If clients complain, don't take it personally, but try to soothe their concerns. Above all, cherish your reputation and respect your clients' feelings and rights. If appointments are running late, anticipate your clients' feelings by informing them ahead of time and asking if they would like some coffee or tea while they're waiting. If a wait is going to be very long, because of an emergency, try to contact clients ahead of time at their homes or offices to avoid displeasure. Be close to long-time clients, but maintain professional integrity.

Remember that education is the best possible teacher. Try to learn from any interactions, whether good or bad, with clients. Be concerned about learning as much as you can about your job; information is the best bond between an esthetician and a skin care client.

SELF-QUIZ: QUESTIONS TO CONSIDER

*Is being a receptionist in a skin care salon good preparation
for a job as a facialist?*

Author's Advice: It certainly can be. A receptionist should be knowledgeable about as many of the services provided at the salon as possible, so that she or he can help explain them to potential clients and arrange for appointments or additional services that complement one another. Many receptionists, in fact, are estheticians who have just graduated from school; because they lack hands-on experience in skin care, they may start as receptionists and then work up to jobs as facialists or, eventually, even managers of salons.

It is important to realize that a receptionist's position is literally that of a front-line representative of the salon. As the first contact with potential clients, the receptionist can make or break a person's impression of the business. A receptionist who is warm and enthusiastic, who answers phones promptly and greets clients warmly, and who helps them feel comfortable in the salon is a highly prized member of a salon's staff.

*I am very interested in skin care but not overly enthusiastic
about makeup. Do I have to wear makeup to succeed in the
beauty business?*

Author's Advice: Although it is possible to succeed in any business through hard work and diligence, the beauty field is a very appearance-conscious world. Even in a skin care salon, most personnel wear at least a little bit of makeup, of the kind that looks as natural as possible but provides a finished appearance. Few women past their twenties can really carry off a totally bare face unless their skin is flawlessly smooth.

That's not to say that you must wear full face makeup to look appropriate. A touch of foundation to smooth out skin tone, a bit of undereye concealer to brighten eye color, and a neutral lip gloss may be all that's needed. Of course, individual salons may have different styles, depending on where they're located, but the amount of makeup you choose to wear should never be the basis on which your job performance is evaluated.

CHAPTER 13   So You Want to Open Your Own Salon?

At some point in many an esthetician's career, the thought arises that having one's own salon would be the ultimate expression of career success. After all, you say to yourself, I know as much about giving facials as my boss and yet the boss is getting all the glory. I'd like to see my name on the door—or on the products I helped develop ideas for selling. The reality, of course, is that there is a lot more to opening and running one's own salon than simply giving facials. A staggering number of small businesses of every kind fail within their first year of operation. Although no one can give you a formula for guaranteed success, there are some important things to consider ahead of time when you think about going into business for yourself. In this chapter, you will find information on:

- defining the market and choosing a location
- regulations and insurance: getting educated (and why your best allies will be your lawyer and your accountant)
- the financial realities: a blueprint of sorts
- planning the salon's layout
- being a good boss and building a strong staff at the same time—and why to do it carefully *and* gradually
- effective advertising and public relations
- building a loyal clientele from the start
- setting prices for services
- opening more than one salon.

DOES THIS NEIGHBORHOOD NEED A NEW SALON?

No matter how wonderful your services, no one will come to a salon if it is not convenient to places of work, business, and shopping. Anyone who plans to open a salon of her own should spend a good deal of time scouting all available spaces in the town and surrounding area. What you want is an attractive space in an active business neighborhood, near department stores, restaurants, and an office building or suburban office park, perhaps. Though it is best to avoid too much competition right nearby (you don't want another skin care salon right in the next building, for example), don't be afraid of an area that already has a salon—that indicates there is a market for these services in the community.

In a city, of course, separating competing businesses by as little as a few blocks is a common strategem. In any town, though, you will want to make a study of the area's demographics to see if there is likely to be a good group of potential clients.

- What is the median income and buying power of the population?
- Are there white-collar workers nearby?
- Are there hotels that draw out-of-town guests who might take advantage of your services?
- Are there exclusive shops nearby?
- Do other business owners in the area think that a skin care salon would be accepted or welcomed?

When looking for an actual space, be on your guard. Few commercial spaces are set up to be salons, and not every space can accommodate one. It's wise to go through a commercial real estate broker, but don't blindly depend on a broker to ask all the right questions. You need to ask as much as possible and to have a lawyer who represents *you*. Not every building is equipped for the additional sinks and plumbing needed for a salon operation, nor does every landlord agree to the open-six-days-a-week policy many salons would like to have (even if you don't plan on this in the beginning, you may want to expand your hours later, so ask). You need an agreement with the landlord that your business hours can be longer than the standard nine to five, as you may want to open early for specific services or stay open late one or more nights a week. In real estate, many people who are eager to rent out space will act as if anything is possible. It's best to have a lawyer see that none of the changes you are planning, either in the arrangement of the space or the hours of operation of your business, would violate any pre-existing zoning codes. You also need to be aware of the **sanitary code** of the city and state to be sure that the salon is arranged in accordance with it. You must, of course, adhere to restrictions on the types of services offered, so that you do not violate medical-practice laws regarding diagnosis or treatment of illnesses. If people will drive to your place of business, you need to check into parking arrangements, whether the parking areas are lit at night, whether you can offer reserved spots for your clients, and so on. Compromises always have to be made when choosing a salon space, and only each individual can decide which are the right choices for her particular business.

A most important consideration in having a **lease** drawn up is that all exceptions to usual business patterns be included within the legal document you will be signing—and that there be specifications as to the alterations that will be made to the space and who will pay for these alterations. Before starting on any costly **renovations**, find out what types of architectural plans must be approved by the local village or city, and be sure to get the necessary approvals before any work is begun. Be wary of **contractors** who balk at waiting or who demand payment ahead of time. Under many agreements, for example, the landlord and the salon owner will split the cost of needed renovations; often, the salon does not pay rent, or pays a greatly reduced monthly fee while the renovations are being done. In a recession or a slow real estate market, obviously, more generous deals are made, but it is still customary for a certain amount of customization of the space to be paid for by the landlord. There should be stipulations within the lease about access to the building by contractors during the renovation; you don't want to suddenly discover that work can only be done after regular business hours, for example. Because of these specific needs, always have a lawyer represent you in leasing arrangements. It's one thing to act on your own when you're renting an apartment; it's another when the lease is for a very specific type of business.

The question arises, of course, of whether one should try to simply take over or buy a share in an ongoing salon business. Many people explore and decide upon that option. Even if a salon already occupied a given space, though, you may want to customize it still further for your needs, for instance, by having fewer or more treatment rooms, smaller or larger space for a reception area, or spaces for manicures, pedicures, and body treatments. Rarely does a salon set up by someone else seem absolutely perfect for your needs.

If there was a salon in the space, but it has gone out of business, an all-important question to explore is *why* the salon failed. Although you may never be able to get a completely accurate answer, it's important to investigate in the neighboring shops to get some educated opinions. The most common reason for salon failures, as with all small businesses, is a lack of **capital** to follow through until profits come in, but that isn't the only reason for a salon to close. Consider the following reasons:

- Were the prices for services too high for the income of the area?
- Was the salon not posh enough for an elitist crowd?
- Were services poorly performed?
- Were the hours of operation not right for the needs of potential clients?
- Do people in this community really understand the need for skin care services? If not, then you might be better off reconsidering the location and opening your own salon somewhere else.

RULES AND REGULATIONS: THE NEED FOR PROFESSIONAL HELP

As already mentioned, a lawyer's advice is greatly beneficial in negotiating a commercial lease. It's also important in setting up a structure for your business, whether you go it alone or take in partners. There are basically three ways to set up a business: as an individual owner, as a corporation or a partnership, or buying into a pre-existing business.

The Individual Owner

An individual owner, or **proprietor**, bears all losses and reaps all profits. However, in a partnership, two or more people pool their resources and expertise, and each partner assumes unlimited liability for losses and draws a predetermined percentage of the profits (most partnerships are even splits if both partners work full-time in the salon; otherwise, an increased compensation is arranged for the partner who will be devoting his or her work time to the salon).

The Corporation

In a **corporation**, an individual or group holds stock in the company, for which a charter is drawn up and a board of directors appointed, with no individual liable for the losses. Although this last may sound like the ideal, there are important legal differences to each business form—and the taxes and fees payable—that a lawyer and/or accountant should be consulted about.

If you are considering incorporating, you must decide what your own individual **total investment** will be, how much you will need others to invest, and how you will apportion the shares of the corporation. Following are examples that will aid you in your decision:

- You might want outside investors to give you a certain amount of capital that would be for stock purchase in addition to a certain amount that would be a loan.

- You would need to present your potential **stockholders** with a three-year projection of sales, profits, and returns on their investment.

- You would need to detail precisely what you will be contributing, not only in terms of money, but also time, expertise, equipment, packaging design, and salon layout plans, for example.

- You would have to itemize the outside capital that you are seeking, in terms of precisely what amounts of money would be used for equipment, furniture, inventory, deposits, advertising or promotion, operating cash, and cash reserve.

- You would need to outline the projected monthly expenses, number of employees, and their salaries and benefit costs, and a realistic accounting of the competition that exists within your community.

It is not easy to obtain outside financing from private individuals or venture-capital groups, but an accountant can give you a good idea of what the current situation is, both nationally and locally. If you are lucky enough to have friends or family—or friends of your family—who are interested in investing, that is often a good place to start. However, be certain that you draw up the same specific business plans that you would for total strangers. Think hard before you go into business with family or friends—there are countless tales of relationships gone sour when a business didn't go exactly as planned. Know your own personality and that of your relatives before you begin.

The Pre-Existing Business

When someone buys a pre-existing salon, there is, in legal parlance, "a transfer of chattel," for which detailed papers of sale must be drawn up (usually by the seller's attorney) and checked carefully for you by legal experts. You should get a complete statement of the inventory, equipment, and furnishings and their true value; the correct identity of all owners; all **liens** against the business; a true representation of the value of the business; an agreement on the use of the current salon name for a defined period of time (this can be in perpetuity if you do not wish to change the name of a successful enterprise); and a guarantee that the seller will not compete with the former business for a set period of time within a certain distance of the salon (a **noncompetition covenant**).

SPOTLIGHT
....

Thirteen years ago, I had a dream: to start my own business. I was eager, over-ambitious, in a rush to be on my own, and woefully ignorant of financial and legal matters. I prepared a business plan on my own and thought that the money would just rush in. The reality was that, after applying to ten different financial institutions all claiming to be interested in helping small businesses—including the U.S. government's Small Business Administration—I got nothing but rejections. I was a woman with no past business experience and no credentials as far as these bankers were concerned. It seemed that one already had to have owned a business in order to get financing for a new one! My work experience counted for nothing. Not a single penny of financing was offered to me.

I started to look into private partners. An acquaintance of mine suggested a woman who had had her own hairstyling salon for ten years. She wanted to expand into other areas and this acquaintance felt we would make a great team. I had knowledge and experience in skin care, makeup, electrolysis, and, especially, in treating male skin care clients. The hairstylist had money to invest and a track record of business ownership. We teamed up, each putting in a small amount of our own money, and against her collateral took out a loan of $150,000. According to the contract, we were 50/50 partners, and if we couldn't meet our payments to the bank, each partner had the right to begin buying shares from the other partner.

We built a beautiful salon in the heart of New York City. I naively accepted her suggestions to get the best of everything—the fanciest flooring, chandeliers, and furniture. In retrospect, we could have spent one-fourth the amount and had a beautiful salon. I went along with my partner's determination to have the best.

It was up to me to run the salon. I hired a staff, trained them, and worked from sunup to sundown to do everything I could to make the place a success. And it was. Within six months, we were breaking even, an amazing feat. I was suddenly in demand for interviews, was in eight different publications in two months, in newspapers, on local television and radio. The only problem was that my partner hadn't planned on this. In fact, she had expected us to do so poorly that she would be able to learn enough about skin care to run the salon on her own and quickly buy me out. She became incredibly jealous that I was getting all the attention from the press. One morning, I arrived at the salon only to find that I had been locked out. The locks had been changed and there was a twenty-four-hour guard there with instructions not to let me on the premises. She told clients or press people looking for me that I was on vacation.

I was devastated. I didn't know where to turn, I had no money for a lawyer, and I barely had the cash to pay my next month's rent for my apartment. With the help of a close friend, I pulled myself together and, with a very short-term loan from another friend, managed to rent a small space in an office building and open my own salon under my name. A newspaper editor who had heard the story of my lockout from a friend wrote a full-page article about my new salon, and within six weeks I made $6,000. Two years later, I had the money to afford a lawyer, who sued my former partner and recovered my money. Within another year, she was forced to close.

People to whom I tell this story usually feel sorry for me, but as an entrepreneur it was the best education ever. It rid me of all my naivete and made me smarter and stronger, since I was able to get up and start over again. I never wasted time being angry, because I literally did not have the time. I had bills to pay, no one else to depend on, and a will to survive. The most important lesson I learned was to be wary of business types who try to take advantage of others.

Another important consideration within any lease agreement, especially if you are taking over a pre-existing salon, is to secure exemptions for fixtures and appliances attached to the store, so that you can remove them at any point without violating your lease. You may not want to undertake the expense of redecorating the space at the outset, but there may come a time when you want to in the future—and you don't want to make elaborate plans only to find out that redoing the space will put you in violation of your lease.

FINANCIAL REALITIES: A BLUEPRINT OF COSTS

Although every business is unique, certain estimates can be made according to industry experience. With an accountant, draw up an estimated financial report. Refer to the following example:

Percentage of Expenses

Salaries	47 percent
Rent	20 percent
Stock and supplies	7 percent
Advertising	3 percent
Electricity/Gas	1 percent

(cont.)

Percentage of Expenses (cont.)

Phone	1 percent
Cleaning	1 percent
Upkeep/Repairs	1.5 percent
Insurance	1.5 percent
Miscellaneous	1 percent
TOTAL	84 percent
PROFIT	16 percent

Of course, these percentages will not bear out during the first year or so, when you may not have any money to spend on professional advertising but will have expenses (to have brochures printed up, etc.) that go beyond 1 percent of the money you take in—and when your profit may well be a loss! That is why you must have a well-capitalized plan, whether based on your own savings or a business loan from family or a bank, before you go into business.

Along with the expenses of leasing space, buying furniture and cabinets, and having telephone lines and utilities installed and maintained, there is the expense of buying supplies. Everything from cotton balls to facial toner and steam equipment must be paid for—and there will be days when the phone may ring only once.

NOTE: Try to arrange a sixty-day credit line with your suppliers so that you don't have to pay for everything up-front.

A strong emotional base is as important as a sound financial one. Be realistic. Better to pay an accountant to draw up a plan for you and find that it may not work after all, and just be out the accountant's fee, than to go brashly into business for yourself only to close down after six months because you've run out of money.

Insurance

An increasing cost for all businesses today is **insurance**. When employing help, you must comply with both local (city and state) and federal laws. **Federal laws** cover social security payments, unemployment insurance payments, and some liability matters. **State law** covers workers' compensation insurance, state taxes, and licenses. **Income taxes** are covered under both state and federal statutes. In addition, of course, a business must have fire, burglary, and theft insurance. Whether you choose to offer health insurance and life insurance to your employees is a matter of choice, but few small businesses can afford to unless government assistance becomes available.

Keeping the Books: Is an Accountant Right for You?

To operate your business properly, you must, of course, keep proper records. You need a **state resale number** to sell beauty products within the salon. If you are set up as a corporation, you must have a **corporate seal** to open a bank account under the business's name. If there are any names—from the name of your salon to the names of particular treatments or products—that you would like to have **trademarked**, you must apply to the trademark authorities in Washington, D.C. There are goods and services taxes, and resale taxes to be paid on any services offered or products sold. A rundown like this shows you why an accountant's advice is a must. In starting out, you should budget in an accountant's consultancy fee for setting up your books for you, even if you cannot afford regular services by a professional bookkeeper and accountant.

SALON LAYOUT: A MATTER OF PRACTICAL DESIGN

If there's one thing we all learn by the time we're adults, it's that everyone has different tastes. What looks like a beautiful house to one person, for example, can be an overdone horror to another. So, although there's no question that interior design can never please everyone all the time, it's also essential that a skin care salon be designed to please as many people as possible, to make clients (and staff) feel comfortable, and to offend no one. What matters the most is clean, neat decor.

Cleanliness is crucial, both for sanitary reasons and for the positive impression it creates. What that means is that the salon should be designed with ease of cleanliness in mind. You should favor surfaces that can be wiped clean, fixtures with a minimum of ornamentation (cut glass, for example, shows a good deal more dust than smooth Plexiglass), and colors that are fresh and bright-looking. You want a layout that uses the space for maximum efficiency and has an ease of flow from room to room, so that you and your staff aren't constantly running back and forth to find things and so that the clients can be quietly led from the reception area to the appropriate treatment rooms. Clean restrooms, adequate air-conditioning and heating systems, and good plumbing and lighting are essentials. Furniture should be well-designed and spare, not overly ornate. The reception area deserves special attention, because it is the source of each client's first impression. If a reception area immediately makes clients feel comfortable, it sends the message that this salon cares about the comfort of everyone who comes through the door.

Whether you choose to work with a professional interior designer or architect or plan the layout of the salon on your own is a matter of personal choice, and may be dictated by how much money you have available. In general, the most practical layouts feature a reception area in which there is ample seating, tables, and an appointment desk adjacent to a display area for product display and sales. The office is then immediately adjacent to the appointment desk. Facial and massage rooms can open off a central hallway, with one additional room set aside for storage of supplies and stock retail items, as well as a laundry room with washer and dryer. A separate room may be set aside for makeup lessons and application, or, if space is at a premium, a makeup area can be set up on one side of the reception area, with lighted mirrors and display cabinets. One rule of thumb: You can never build too many cabinets—in the individual treatment rooms, in the storage room, and in the office area. There is always a need to have supplies on hand and the more they are kept out of sight, the neater and more appealing the salon will look.

Security and Safety

The reality of modern life is that security and safety have to be part of the salon layout. Many modern-day security systems have a direct link to the police department; if you are in an urban area or any area in which crime is a problem, this is a must and well worth the monetary expense for your own peace of mind. Any system, of course, is only good if people know how to use it. Be sure to teach all your employees what to do in an emergency, where the buttons are, where the fire exits are, and so on. Fire drills should be conducted every six months, and always when new employees are hired. (Though this point sounds childishly obvious, it is incredible how often it is overlooked.) Your employees must know where all the safety exits are so that they do not panic in case of any emergency, but can help each other and the clients to safe passage from the building should any type of problem occur.

Every salon should also have a **first-aid kit** on hand to treat any small injuries that occur. This kit should include adhesive bandages, sterile cotton, antibiotic cream, antiseptic cleanser or alcohol pads, sterile bandages, and first-aid tape. Of course, if anyone is badly injured, everyone should know to call 911 or the local equivalent.

BEING A GOOD BOSS—AND BUILDING YOUR STRONG STAFF GRADUALLY

One of the biggest changes most people make when starting a business of their own is in becoming the boss. Even if you were the manager of a salon for years, you still reported, ultimately, to the salon ownership. Now, for the first time ever, you will live by the motto "the buck stops here." If things go well, you can take a lot of pride in them, but when problems occur, it is you who must smooth things out. One of the most delicate issues of all is dealing with employees. The first decision to be made is whether to hire anyone at all when you first start out.

The Hiring Process

Being careful about hiring is a skill unto itself, as is knowing whom to hire and being a good boss. Obviously, you want people with experience, a love of the business, and personalities that will mesh with yours and your type of clientele. Even with all these guidelines, though, it comes down to a judgment call in the end. But don't have overly high expectations: you need to train *every* new employee, regardless of experience, in your own techniques and preferred way of providing services to clients within your salon. You need to give employees positive feedback for jobs well done as well as constructive criticism for things that could be done better. One golden rule: Never criticize employees in front of clients. Have these conversations in private, so that you don't risk having a perfectly satisfactory staff member who simply made a mistake quit due to embarrassment.

Though opinions differ, it is often wise to have employees sign some sort of agreement about their conduct within the salon and what they may do should they leave to work for a competitor. There is no magic formula for successful relations between bosses and employees, but a written contract does make certain points absolutely clear. If you do want to draw up such a **contract**, of course, it is wise to go over it with a lawyer to be sure that the language is legally correct. Here are some items that are often included in such a contract:

- a term of service, usually running for one year, unless terminated by either party

- termination notice, specifying two weeks for either being fired or quitting

- salary, bonuses, and lists of duties and responsibilities (these can be as general as "attention to the business of Sally Mae Skin Care Salon" or more specific and detailed listings). If a commission is offered on the sale of products, such as moisturizers or nail polishes, it should be specified.

- schedule of performance reviews and reimbursement (if any) for use of car, entertainment, educational expenses

- specifics of health and insurance plans, as well as vacation schedules, sick days, and (if allowed) personal days.

Such a contract does not, of course, preclude there being any discussion of specific issues that differ from the standard contract, but it can be a good starting point and an indication of professionalism on the salon's part. Similar contracts may be drawn up with those working as independent contractors within the salon. (This is often done for part-time personnel, such as electrologists or masseuses, for example, who may work at different salons on different days of the week.)

The emphasis on being a good boss invariably involves matters such as supervision, teaching, and reviewing employees' performance, but it is important to remember that we are all human beings. One of the most common mistakes that inexperienced managers make is to overemphasize the distance they must maintain between themselves and their employees. As a result, they can be cold and ever on the alert, out of a fear of being taken advantage of, with the result that employees don't feel comfortable airing their views and work in fear rather than in pleasure. In such an atmosphere, nobody, boss or staff, does the best possible work. It's a good idea to establish communication with your staff early on; although you don't need (or want) to become best friends with your employees, it is important that they know they can come to you with ideas, complaints, suggestions, and problems so that you can help them make the salon a pleasant place to work.

GETTING THE WORD OUT: EFFECTIVE ADVERTISING AND PUBLIC RELATIONS

The first, most effective method of advertising may come as a surprise to you: it is the look and atmosphere of your salon and the professionalism of everyone involved with it. No advertising campaign in the world will bring you success if the salon itself is dark or dingy or clients are kept waiting too long for their appointments. So before you commit a cent to advertising, be sure the salon itself is presented professionally.

How would you spread the word about the salon's grand opening? The best way is to start planning ahead of time by assembling a list of friends, relatives, acquaintances, and personal contacts to whom to send announcements two weeks before the grand opening. One thing you may be tempted to do is begin with a list of former clients, but this is *definitely not professionally correct.* It is one thing to inform certain clients that you will be heading out in business alone, but to try to woo them away from a former place of your employment is very indiscreet. (To understand why, simply imagine yourself in the same situation as your former business's owner!) Don't worry; once the word spreads that you have left the salon to go out on your own, your most loyal clients will find you.

How to get the word spread without spending a fortune is, of course, a challenge. First of all, try to get as much **free publicity** as you can. This is not only important when your business first opens but is, in fact, the way to remain successful throughout the years. Ask friends and relatives if they know people in the newspaper or magazine business; you may be quite surprised at the contacts you didn't even know you had. Then send those contacts announcements of the salon's opening, any unique services you will be offering, or special promotional offers you have planned. Do the same for names in the newspapers and magazines who write about the subjects of fashion or beauty. Include a short biography of yourself and your experience and training with the press announcement. Don't be shy about who you send it to, and try to follow up with phone calls if you can. Remember, the news media are looking for news, and you can provide it.

Another good way to get people to try your salon is to print up **gift certificates** for half-price services and offer to sell them to anyone who comes in, to pass along to friends, clients, or family. Have an open-house-style grand opening and try to invite any "newsworthy" people you know, whether they are local community government officials or other notables—then invite the press to cover the event. Target twenty people in newspapers, twenty in television, and twenty in radio or magazines to receive your mailings and send each one an invitation to visit the salon at his or her convenience. Contact the concierges at nearby hotels and invite them to visit the salon; they can then give firsthand information on the services you offer to visitors. Let local modeling agencies know about your opening, as they often send aspiring models for facials and other beauty treatments. An important group of professionals not to overlook is dermatologists and plastic surgeons, who should all receive invitations to visit the salon at their convenience. If you start out by dealing with medical professionals as professionals, rather than as adversaries, you can develop quite a nice rapport with them. You may be able to gain referrals for facials, for example, or have someone to call upon should a medical question come up within the context of salon services.

The Problems of Advertising

Advertising is often touted as being the most effective way to let people know about new products and services. Although this is true, it's also expensive, and few people just starting out in business have that much to spend. After all, few of us can write or design our own ads, so we need to be able to pay someone to do that first, and then pay for its placement in the media.

When you are ready to advertise, the question will be where to advertise. Along with many small businesses, skin care salons usually find that the most reasonable place to begin advertising is where people look every day, in the newspapers and telephone book. You might begin with a small ad in a local newspaper along with a listing in the Yellow Pages. Direct-mail advertising is more expensive but is a good next step. Radio is more expensive, but can also be effective if you choose a locally targeted station. Magazines are expensive and television is even more so, although one exception may be local cable television stations that provide help in producing the commercials for small businesses. But these last methods are really something to be looked into down the road, once the business is established.

At every stage of business, don't overlook opportunities to get publicity about your salon for a nominal cost, in a way that will bring potential customers into the salon. You might donate gift certificates to local charities for door prizes or raffles, offer to give lectures/demonstrations at women's club and men's club meetings, participate in public forums, speak at local health clubs, and so on. To this day, there is no ad campaign as effective as being interviewed by the press; it immediately gives you and your salon a legitimacy as a source of valid, useful information. It brings in new clients and lets existing clients get positive reassurance that they are going to a salon that is newsworthy and respected. The effect is often longer lasting than you think; people may clip out an article and not call right away, but arrange an appointment a few months later. Or they may read a magazine from last month, rather than this month, at the beauty salon and make a note of a treatment they want to try.

When individual members of the press do visit the salon, don't make the mistake of giving them a sales pitch. You want to put your best foot forward, but you need to give a reporter a reason to believe that you are a cut above the other salons in your area. This isn't done by self-aggrandizement, but by offering information. Have information sheets ready on the various services offered, and be willing to take time to explain them and give general advice on skin care. Be sure everyone in the salon is aware that a press visitor is there, so that they can be as conscientious as possible. Show members of the press that you are knowledgeable about general skin care questions, not just about the specific services you offer, and they will come back to you with questions for future articles.

ATTRACTING AND KEEPING A LOYAL CLIENTELE

When Mother Nature simply creates a beautiful place, people will come. In the hustle-bustle business world, though, having a nice-looking building isn't enough. You need to give clients a reason to come to you *and* a reason to come back again. The answer, in a word, is **service**.

Salon service starts the moment the phone rings, a fact too few places acknowledge. Modern phone systems may increasingly rely on voice machines, but skin care is a personal business. The person who answers the phone has one of the most important tasks of all. Each phone call is a chance to build a reputation. You need to answer questions in a friendly, informative way, whether you (the owner) are doing the answering in the beginning or having someone else do it for you in the end. Each caller is a potential client who, depending on how she or he is treated, may well decide based on the phone call whether to book an appointment at the salon. Questions may run from how much a basic facial costs to how long a specific service takes to what your hours of business are. If you are running a special promotion, a caller may have a question about that. Patience is a necessity, as some people are less articulate than others; but if you must put someone on hold, be sure to go back to them. If a caller is taking too much of your time at a busy hour, politely explain the situation, take the number, and arrange a time to call back. This is preferable to hurrying them off the phone, which may result in their simply deciding not to visit the salon.

Management experts who have made studies of telephone styles recommend the following four essentials for a positive phone image:

1. **A helpful attitude**. An enthusiastic tone of voice is a big selling point.

2. **Promptness**. Letting the phone ring again and again without anyone answering it will lead some people to hang up in disgust and others to feel that their calls are considered unimportant. Clients already in the salon will also be subjected to the annoying noise. Neither is the result you're after.

3. **Identify the business upon answering**. "LaDiDa Salon, may I help you?" is a more appropriate answer than "Hello, may I help you?"

4. **Inquire who is calling in a polite way**. If someone does not identify herself, but asks a lot of questions, or asks to speak to the manager or owner, the receptionist should ask, nicely, "Whom shall I say is calling?" Then the information being asked for can be clearly passed along to the person the call is intended to reach.

Good planning in business involves assigning the right persons to tasks and giving them the information they need to conduct business. The telephone, for example, should be right near the appointment book, because a big part of phone work in a salon is booking appointments. And proper booking practices can make the difference between success and failure.

Scheduling: The Dilemma of Overbooking

Every service business has a tendency to overbook, despite the fact that this is a key cause of displeasure among customers. Try to resist falling into this trap if at all possible. You know how long a facial lasts—usually fifty minutes—so book each client for a full hour if you are the only one giving facials in the salon. If you have an assistant who performs some portions of the facial, such as skin cleansing and steaming, then you can book a client every half hour. Don't believe anyone who tells you that more is possible. Some salons book clients every fifteen minutes, and then leave them waiting a minimum of fifteen minutes each beyond their appointment time before they are even brought into the facial room. This arrangement may produce extra revenue for a while, but eventually it will backfire, because your clients will not appreciate all that waiting time.

Overbooking also gives you no flexibility when it comes to the reality of how business runs and your and your clients' lives work. If one client is fifteen minutes late, everything else gets thrown off schedule—but the reality is that a client may be caught in a traffic jam or held up in a meeting at work. You may be late one morning, too, through no fault of your own. If a client is fifteen minutes late and has not yet called the salon to let you know, you have every right to start on someone else and then try to work the late client in when she arrives. Some services can be switched around if you have extra rooms and the personnel to do it, but in a small salon, it may be literally impossible to accommodate people who don't show up reasonably on time. Be diplomatic in asking what kept the person and let the client know what arrangements you can make. Similarly, every appointment booking should include an inquiry for a number at which the client can be reached, so that you can let him or her know if you are running far behind. Salons with adequate personnel often call to reconfirm appointments a day ahead, to encourage timeliness.

Aside from keeping everyone running on time and aware of their responsibilities for the day, an appointment book is an important record of the most popular services at the salon. A daily review of the book can help the manager or owner to anticipate what supplies should be ordered, and it can alert an esthetician as to how to schedule an individual client's time if that client is also having additional services during the same salon visit. Additionally, the appointment book will reveal who your "frequent visitor" clients are; these are the clients to whom you may want to offer the convenience of booking special packages of X number of facials at a discount, or X number of facials plus X number of manicures or pedicures, for example. Specific mailings could be made to those who have visited the salon more than five times within a six-month period, for example.

PROMOTIONS Within the salon, promotions are a very underutilized way of keeping clients coming back for more. If the going rate for facials in your community, for example, is $50, and that is the amount you have always charged, you may want to run a "spring cleaning sale" of facials for $45 during the month of May. In fact, you may want to run a special each month to help get your clients to sample new services. Be creative with your ideas. For instance, offer a facial/manicure combination at a discount, or run a special promotion of at-home skin products at a discount if purchased at the time of a facial.

SETTING SALON PRICES: A DELICATE BALANCE

Talk of special discounts inevitably brings up the whole question of salon prices. At one time, especially during the go-go years of the 1980s, it was thought that no prices could be too high for the rich and famous, whom everyone anticipated would come to the trendiest salon regardless of price. Well, in New York City, two very famous hairdressers—featured in all the fashion magazines, interviewed by beauty editors galore—found out the hard way that one can literally price oneself out of business. They both opened lavish salons, decorated them gloriously, and set prices for haircuts sky-high. At first, their bookings were pretty impressive, but then even the rich started having second thoughts about paying twice as much as the most expensive salons charged simply to have their hair cut. Over time, appointments dwindled. One salon lasted roughly one year, the other (because it featured a few more reasonably priced cutters, who had their own followings) about two years. When their doors shut, no one asked why: the prices were simply too high.

Setting prices for typical services involves calculating the costs of the products used, employees' salaries (or the owner's), the basic overhead expenses of the business, and a last factor—ignored at one's own peril: a knowledge of "what the traffic will bear." Even a famous restaurant doesn't charge as much in Chicago as its sister establishment does in New York City, so don't be fooled by what big-city salons do if you're located in Ames, Iowa. One well-recognized way to gain an idea of the range within which to set prices is by checking what the competition currently charges, and then figuring out if the clientele you are aiming at is the same, slightly more upscale, or a bit less affluent. You may choose to match prices on some services but undercut the competition on others. During the first month you are open, for example, you might run a grand opening special during which you cut your planned price on one or two services to encourage customers to give you a try. Many new salons have become successful in areas in which only very pricy establishments existed beforehand, by providing quality treatments in an atmosphere that, though attractive to affluent clients, also appeals to those who desire the services provided by the more opulent salons but at prices they can better afford.

Once prices are set, be wary of raising them too often. For this reason, it's appropriate to run a limited-time offer of lower prices during the first month you are open, but don't extend the discounts for too long. If you do, your clients will feel taken advantage of—you will appear to have waited until they became regulars to raise your prices.

SHOULD YOU OPEN MORE THAN ONE SALON?

In the very beginning, the answer to expansion is no. You should wait five to six years to establish a name for yourself, and learn the true ins and outs of business, before trying to expand. It may seem tempting to turn a fast success into an even bigger one, but expanding too soon can turn a profitable business into a failure. It takes a great deal of energy to run one salon, let alone several, so it really makes sense to firmly establish yourself before you decide on expansion.

Before embarking on an expansion plan, you need to consider the following factors:

- Do you have the financial wherewithal to do it on your own, or will you need outside capital?

- Do you have an employee upon whom you could rely to run the current salon in your absence, or will you need to hire and train someone?

- Do you have a specific location in mind for the new salon?

- Are you ready to commit to the travel involved in regularly commuting between the two locations?

The next step after thinking about these things is to draw up the same type of detailed business plan as you did for starting out (if you didn't do it the first time, then it's definitely a must for any considered expansion). Once you put down on paper what it will really cost to open a second operation, you can better assess whether your current business generates enough cash to finance an expansion or, if not, how much outside capital you will need. With an accountant or lawyer's advice, you can then approach local bank lending officers, venture capital groups, or individual investors. Don't underestimate, though, how much time it can take to find people willing to invest in small businesses. Our society seems to pay a great deal of lip service to the notion of helping small businesses, but many going concerns are routinely turned down for traditional loans. Before you even apply, you must be able to detail exactly how much you need and project the cash flow on a monthly basis, annual basis, and for the first two to three years of expansion. You must also acknowledge and consider the toll it will take on you in terms of time, energy, and money, to be sure that this is the right time for you to expand.

LEARNING FROM EXAMPLE: THE BEST SKIN CARE SALONS

Anyone who is considering opening a salon should have already spent several years working for a top salon, learning by example and absorbing all the information available on a daily basis. It is also a good idea, though, to have visited other salons, for inspiration and ideas and to see how different individuals put their own personal stamp on the business. The truth is that there is no formula for a successful business of any kind, especially a salon, which involves the personal service given and received by unique individuals. Each salon represents the spirit as well as the knowledge of the person who founded it. Each person's approach is different. This is part of the pleasure of the skin care business, because it is a business in which you can invest your own outlook as well as your education and experience.

SELF-QUIZ: QUESTIONS TO CONSIDER

I have a client list of fifty people who always book their facial appointments with me, after just one year of working at a skin care salon. Can't I take these clients with me if I want to open a business on my own?

Author's Advice: This is a very difficult ethical question, but one on which the moral answer is clear: No one should try to steal clients from another business. You should never solicit your customers if you leave, whether to work for someone else or to go out on your own. The advertising for your own salon will draw them (as could ads from your new employer, the reason salons frequently run ads "welcoming so-and-so" to our staff). Actually, it is wrong to truly consider them *your* clients; in fact, they are the clients of the salon for which you work. Some people ignore this distinction, but as a possible future employer, you should recognize that it is wrong.

It also seems a little premature to think about going out on your own. It takes a good two years of working for someone else to truly establish yourself within a field and to take advantage of all there is to learn. Don't rush yourself.

I would love to have a salon of my own, but I'm not very organized about record keeping. Is this a big problem?

Author's Advice: Definitely. If you want to go into business, keeping well-organized records is a necessity. You need a card file system or book to record all services with clients, their names and addresses and phone numbers, what products were used, and what they bought (and if you had any problems with their credit or checks bouncing). You need to keep track of inventory, to prevent running short or overordering. You need to keep daily appointment lists, petty cash books, and daily receipts, not only for current records but for at least a full year. All transactions must be recorded to provide a record of income or loss, to reflect the value of the salon, to comply with wage and hour laws, to have tax records, and so on. Most accountants advise keeping complete records for seven years, the length of time during which one can be audited.

In addition, there is really no other way than having records to review to be able to assess how your business is doing. How will you know what services are most frequently requested? Which ones do you need to promote more or consider discontinuing? How often do your regular clients come in? Those who are unable to keep good records may find that they are also unable to run a business on their own. They might be the best candidates for going into a partnership with someone who is more managerial and administrative-minded.

I've been employed by a top-notch salon for six years, and my husband thinks I'd really be able to make a go of it on my own. But I'm not sure I'm cut out to be a boss. What does it take?

Author's Advice: A good boss is probably nearly impossible to define, but it takes a mixture of toughness and caring, experience and knowledge, as well as an effort to understand and motivate employees. Too much fear of being taken advantage of can make a boss blind to the fact that employees need caring, courtesy, and encouragement. On the other hand, being too much of a friend to one's employees isn't in anyone's best interest either, because professionalism is essential to a good salon operation. In the skin care business, everyone tells the salon owner about their troubles—your clients, your employees, your suppliers. You need to be able to lend an ear when it's essential but not to encourage an overly personal relationship with business colleagues and employees.

Your husband probably knows you better than anyone else, so he must feel that you would be a good entrepreneur for a reason. Ask him what he thinks your strengths are, and compare his list with your own feelings about yourself. One thing is for certain, though. Running one's own business takes a great deal of energy and determination, so it should be a decision one makes for oneself, not because someone else thinks it's a good idea.

CHAPTER 14   Staying on Your Toes

In any field, one of the biggest challenges is to stay on top of the latest developments while still performing at your best. In the skin care profession, this is especially important, because new developments occur at a breakneck pace. As soon as scientists discover some new little fact about the skin, salons race to take advantage of the discovery with a new treatment said to be precisely targeted to this cell or that substance. The search for something new is constant, because every salon is looking for the magic new treatment that will attract new customers and entice more people to try facials or body treatments. In this chapter, you will learn how to:

- stay current and know what organizations and publications can provide new knowledge

- stay one step ahead of your clients, or anticipate their needs as soon as something new hits the market

- keep up your enthusiasm year in and year out

- turn your knowledge into teaching possibilities for the public and the profession.

GROUPS THAT ARE WORTH THE MEMBERSHIP FEE

The number of organizations that can provide information on skin care continues to grow. So does the range of organizations geared to entrepreneurs and/or female business leaders. In many cases, the biggest benefit of these groups is not only what they themselves provide, but the opportunity for **networking** with other professionals. Meeting people in your own profession can help to foster camaraderie rather than competition, and can give you a chance to learn about salon services in other parts of the country and other parts of the world. Some groups sponsor workshops that can inspire new ideas; others can link you with people in your area who have specific knowledge and expertise (for example, you may need help in locating a licensed massage therapist to refer clients to, or to hire for a salon). Here are some of the groups that have proven worthwhile. *This is by no means an exhaustive list; there may be other organizations that are also valuable.*

- *Aesthetics International Association (AIA)*
  4447 McKinney Avenue
  Dallas, TX 75205
  (214) 526-0752

- *American Women's Economic Development Corporation (AWED)*
  71 Vanderbilt Avenue
  New York, NY 10017
  (212) 692-9100

- *Cosmetic Executive Women*
  217 East 85th Street, Suite 214
  New York, NY 10028
  (212) 759-3283

- *Cosmetic, Toiletries and Fragrances Association (CTFA)*
  1101 17th Street NW, Suite 300
  Washington, DC 20036
  (202) 331-1770

- *Fashion Group, Inc.*
  597 5th Avenue
  New York, NY 10017
  (212) 593-1715

- *National Association of Female Executives (NAFE)*
  127 West 24th Street, 4th Floor
  New York, NY 10011
  (212) 645-0770

- *Reflexology Institute*
  P.O. Box 12642
  St. Petersburg, FL 33733
  (813) 343-4811

- *Society of Cosmetic Chemists (SCC)*
  1995 Broadway, Suite 1701
  New York, NY 10022
  (212) 874-0600

- *Swedish Massage Institute*
  226 West 26th Street, 5th Floor
  New York, NY 10001
  (212) 924-5900

STAYING AHEAD OF THE PACK

The only way to stay in business, survive, and help to spread information about the business of skin care is to stay one step ahead of the competition. The first way to stay on top of what's new is literally to read the news. That means not only reading the day's newspapers (most of which do have a "style" or "women's" page, which can offer tidbits of new ideas) but also, once every week, glancing through all the beauty publications. When you first start out, you should read everything in these magazines from cover to cover. There is no better way to glean ideas on everything from the way to set up your salon, to how to promote it, to how to continue to expand the services you offer. As you progress through the years, you can skim parts of the magazines that cover those things you already feel expert on, but concentrate more on articles describing new types of facials, body treatments, or hair and scalp treatments. You should literally look for news from everywhere—cosmetic chemists, editors, retail establishments, and so on.

Another source of new ideas, of course, is the **trade shows** that are held once a year in major cities across the United States. Many are sponsored by trade magazines or industry groups. Just be aware that you don't have to buy anything at these shows. A good deal of hype and heavy-handed salesmanship goes on, so prepare yourself ahead of time to be an educated consumer. Collect all the brochures, leaflets, and business cards you can and then review them in the quiet and privacy of your own office at home. Don't let anyone talk you into signing up for a huge delivery of creams or lotions that you don't even have a precise use for yet. Also, don't overlook the value of going to gain new ideas even if you don't have money to spend right now. Better to be educated ahead of time and then to have the information available to you once you are in a position to order new supplies.

Similarly, don't overlook the chance whenever you travel, for business or pleasure, to get new ideas from local salons and local magazines and newspapers (or just from local customs). Attend lectures whenever possible. Try things out yourself; if they're not worthwhile, you'll learn so firsthand.

As soon as you read or hear about something new that sounds valuable or worthwhile, research it by checking in other trade magazines for information. Then ask beauty-product suppliers if it's something they offer. If it is, consider ordering a small amount and trying the treatment yourself, or using it on a salon staff member to see how it works. If it's all that's promised, introduce it in the salon. Even with the most fantastic new treatment, though, don't necessarily expect it to be an overnight hit. This may come as a shock within a business that seems to thrive on new and improved products and processes, but it takes about two years to truly saturate a market with an idea. There will be a small group of clients who want to try anything new immediately, but many will wait for their friends to try it, to read more about it, and to see results in someone else.

Whenever you decide to introduce something new, don't give up on it too fast. Everything that is introduced in a quality salon should be kept on as a service, not thrown away once it's no longer new. Once your clients see benefits from a treatment, they don't want to give it up just because it is no longer making headlines in a magazine. Remember, it will take a full two years for the majority of your salon clients to have sampled a new procedure.

In fact, one of the biggest mistakes some salons make is constantly latching onto new services while neglecting the tried-and-true. The bottom line with new offerings is that your clients will try them based on their trust and long-term relationship with you. Once they have seen the benefits, for example, of a year or more of basic facials, they may want to give something else a chance. What they are expressing is a trust in you to prove to them again that you can make their skin still better than it is already. If you constantly churn the services you offer by discarding what works for something new every other month, you will disappoint your most loyal and faithful clients who have come to depend on you.

Keeping Your Staff Up-to-Date

It is of no benefit at all if the salon's owner or manager is the only one who is knowledgeable about the latest trends and treatments. Every staff member should be given as much continuing education as possible. Whenever new services are offered, training sessions should be arranged for the entire staff (it's a smart idea to include even those who don't directly offer services, such as receptionists, so that they can answer any questions clients may have). Take advantage of **training seminars** offered by companies that distribute or manufacture beauty products whenever you can. Beware of companies that don't offer any hands-on training along with the products they sell; an indication of the seriousness of a company is how much it is willing to invest in time and personnel to support the products it sells.

When signing up for workshops offered by trade magazines, use the chance to offer this as a special perquisite for salon staffers (in fact, many seminars offer some type of group discount, so look into this as well).

A staff that is involved in this way can be a strong source of new ideas. Once they know that the salon management is interested in their training and knowledge, they will feel free to come forward with their own ideas as well.

Continuing seminars and meetings among the staff can help not only in keeping everyone current but also in airing any problems or questions staffers have. This can keep any resentment from developing. It is also a chance to let everyone see the brochures or leaflets that have been prepared in advance of offering new treatments, so that the entire staff knows what is being promoted at the moment.

ENTHUSIASM: HOW TO KEEP IT GOING AND GROWING

The biggest question for a skin care professional is how to keep your spirit, emotion, and intensity and still stay enthusiastic and passionate about your work. For the lucky among us, it comes naturally, but, as in a good marriage or family, it's a type of caring that also takes hard work and sacrifice. As wonderful as it is to be in a business you love, it is constantly demanding of time, effort, and energy. You need to remember that everyone has to be "refueled" now and then. When you're lucky, that means taking a vacation. When you're not that fortunate at that time, it can mean just taking a Sunday to laze around the house and do nothing more than read the newspaper, play with your child, chat with an old friend, or do anything that takes your mind completely off your work. Another valuable type of regeneration is to stay as informed as possible about new ideas, to take each step of building your own reputation and your business one step at a time, to take a moment now and then to take stock of (and pride in) what you have accomplished, and to share that enthusiasm with the other workers within the salon.

One suggestion is to gather together all your employees for a meeting (try starting out once every two to three weeks) to remind them that they are in a salon in which much more than the basics are offered. Following is a sample agenda that may help in the early stages:

- Talk about what's newest in makeup trends, nail colors, treatments and services.

- Offer a small pep talk on how well you feel the staff is doing and what you need to promote at the moment.
- If there's a new spring makeup palette, discuss ways to tell clients about it, through in-salon posters, half-price makeup lessons, or whatever.
- Ask for suggestions, so everyone feels involved.

Emphasize that there are no rules at these meetings; everyone should feel free to come forward with ideas. It's a time for what corporations call "blue-sky ideas," meaning that you can suggest something as high as the sky. It's a chance to focus not only on the here-and-now of everyday business realities, but also to express enthusiasm about the future. In times of economic downturn, when things might not be going as well as you hoped, it's a chance to be honest with everyone and map out a plan to help build business. When times are stressful, this type of meeting can be an important way for people to vent their worries and, hopefully, feel reinvigorated about brighter possibilities ahead.

At this meeting, also let employees know if the salon is involved in any projects at the management level, such as a donation of gift certificates to a charity raffle, so that they know potential new clients may be coming in soon. The staff can also suggest other causes to you that you may not be aware of, so that you can continue to spread goodwill throughout your community.

SPREADING THE WORD: USING YOUR KNOWLEDGE TO TEACH OTHERS AND BUILD YOUR NAME

During the first five years of any salon business, there is a golden opportunity not only to build a business but also to teach oneself, as a professional, how to teach others. Too often, people don't even realize their own potential as a spokesperson because they never give public speaking a try. When yours is a relatively new business, this can also be a way to introduce yourself to others within the community who may not be aware of your establishment. As with any new endeavor, it is wise to start small.

The first rule of **public speaking** is to let people know you are available. Look into adult education programs sponsored by the local high school first, for example. Call them up and volunteer to teach a class on at-home skin care for adults. It could be a one-session program, if you wish, or a series of workshops. To get yourself started, don't even ask for a fee; just volunteer your time. Other places to call are local modeling

SPOTLIGHT

My first series of lectures to the public was at The Learning Annex in New York City and came about quite by chance. This organization, which sponsors continuing education classes for adults in several major cities across the country, had just started, and they were as inexperienced as I was. I had always dreamed of being a teacher when I was younger, but I didn't see much chance of fulfilling that dream once I was in my own business—especially since I was just starting out, in my first year on my own.

As fate would have it, though, I hired a woman as a facialist whose brother-in-law was also an entrepreneur and had just come up with the idea of The Learning Annex. She didn't work for me for very long, as she decided to quit soon after becoming pregnant, but she referred her brother-in-law to me and told him I knew everything about skin care, especially for men. He came up with the idea of offering two sets of classes, one for men and one for women, on skin care. When he contacted me, I was so flattered that I didn't have the nerve to tell him I'd never spoken in front of a group before.

I spent two weeks preparing for my first class for men. I rewrote what I was going to say a hundred times, at least, and prepared bags full of products to bring along to demonstrate, along with books and brochures. To say I was nervous is a massive understatement; it was all I could do to look up at the class of eight men and begin talking. But once I began, I saw that they were all actually interested in what I had to say. After the second class, my confidence began to grow. What had taken me two weeks to prepare at first now took me five days; then, eventually, two. From that first group of classes—eight men and about a dozen women—my classes eventually became one of the most popular offerings. One semester, I had almost fifty women sign up for my class. The secret, I found, whatever the size of the group, was to try to get them involved in the subject on a personal level. The best technique was not just to trot out my technical knowledge, but to ask for volunteers within the class to demonstrate—whether it was analyzing several people's skin, asking people to feel the difference in "weight" between various creams, or asking them to describe their own personal skin care routines. I learned that I couldn't just be a distant teacher in these classes; I had to be, in essence, a missionary for skin care.

Over time, I went on to speak to bigger audiences and various professional groups. I always ask an audience to interrupt at any time with questions—to remember that I know what I know, but I don't know what they want to learn about. Today, fifteen years after my first lecture, I still remember my initial nervousness but now know that feeling comfortable with the subject of skin care means that I can eventually feel comfortable speaking about it in front of any type of group.

I also learned an important lesson from one of my earliest lectures: Don't be concerned about speaking fees; just be willing to share your knowledge. You never know who will be in the audience. In one of my free lectures, there was a whole group of magazine editors in the audience. After I told my story of starting my own business with barely any money at all, two of the editors approached me after my lecture. It turned out they wanted to include me in major feature articles about struggling to start a business. What had started out as an unpaid speaking date turned into the type of national magazine publicity I could never afford to buy.

agencies, who are often delighted to have guest lecturers come in and speak to their students—models are, after all, seeking to be in the forefront of the appearance business. Women's organizations in the community are also always looking for guest speakers at their monthly or bimonthly meetings, so call up, introduce yourself as a new business in town, and ask to speak to the person who arranges guest lectures. If you prove to have a talent for leading these discussions, the word will spread and other groups will contact you. In addition, when members of the audience are considering professional skin care treatment, they will remember you as someone knowledgeable in the field and will be more likely to consider your salon.

If you are offering a public workshop of some kind, it also makes sense to send out a **press release** to local newspapers or radio shows. They might want to publicize the event ahead of time or even send a reporter to cover the program. Again, this is a way to spread knowledge about the skin care field while also enhancing your own reputation and expanding your field of contacts within the community.

SELF-QUIZ: QUESTIONS TO CONSIDER

I am a beauty-school student and recently attended a beauty trade show in the capital of my state. I was shocked at the hard-sell techniques used for some of the treatments; one company promised that its product was "equal to a face-lift." Is this possible?

Author's Advice: Of course it is not possible for any cosmetic treatment to be equal to a face-lift—no cream can perform surgery. But the trend you point to is a strong one. Beauty companies are promising more and more, sometimes going so far as such extreme exaggerations as the one you heard. The goal of trade shows is, after all, to sell products to the trade—beauty salons, skin care salons, and retail establishments. Some of the sales techniques used can, unfortunately, be terribly over hyped.

That doesn't mean that trade shows aren't valuable, though. Not every booth will feature a hard-sell technique, and many of the products are very worthwhile. For a student, it is a good education to see the gamut of offerings in equipment and products, and to start to learn to separate the honest from the not-so-honest in the profession. Even established businesspeople often go to trade shows more for a "look-see" than to buy. It's always a great place to learn about the latest advances, pick up brochures and contacts about new offerings, and take home as many samples and booklets as possible to review in the privacy of one's own salon. Frequently, the things you see at the trade show turn out to be items you would like to purchase in the future, and you have already made the initial contact with the company representative ahead of time.

The salon where I work is always offering new treatments, but frequently discontinues them after a year. Is this a smart move?

Author's Advice: Giving one's clientele only a year to sample new treatments seems a little shortsighted. It generally takes about two years to saturate a market with a new idea, to give everyone a chance to sample a new treatment. Keep in mind that there will always be a group of clients who immediately want to try something new and then, after a few months, are eager for the next new, improved offering. But there are many people who want to think about something for a while, hear about results from others, read about skin care ideas in magazines, and then at last try the new idea out. If you stop offering it after a year, they may simply miss the chance to try the treatment, and the salon will miss out on the revenue as well. In addition, a year is too short a time to tell if a new treatment should become a standard, something that is offered all the time in the salon for those who want to stick with the benefits.

Our salon is frequently approached by charitable groups for donations. We can't afford to give money to all of these groups. Would giving a discount certificate as a raffle prize be a good idea?

Author's Advice: Giving a gift of salon services is a very worthwhile idea. If you can't afford to give a gift certificate for a specific service, fully paid, however, it may be touchy, because you would be expecting prize winners to supplement the certificates with their own money in order to redeem the prize. Perhaps it would be better to wait until the business is better established and you can afford to give a gift certificate outright as the prize. Don't overlook the option to offer a lower-cost service, such as a manicure or pedicure, as the donation. This is as welcome as a higher-cost facial or body treatment and may give the business the option of being a charitable donor sooner than you expected.

Glossary/Index

Note: Page numbers in **bold** type reference non-text material.